COMMANDO

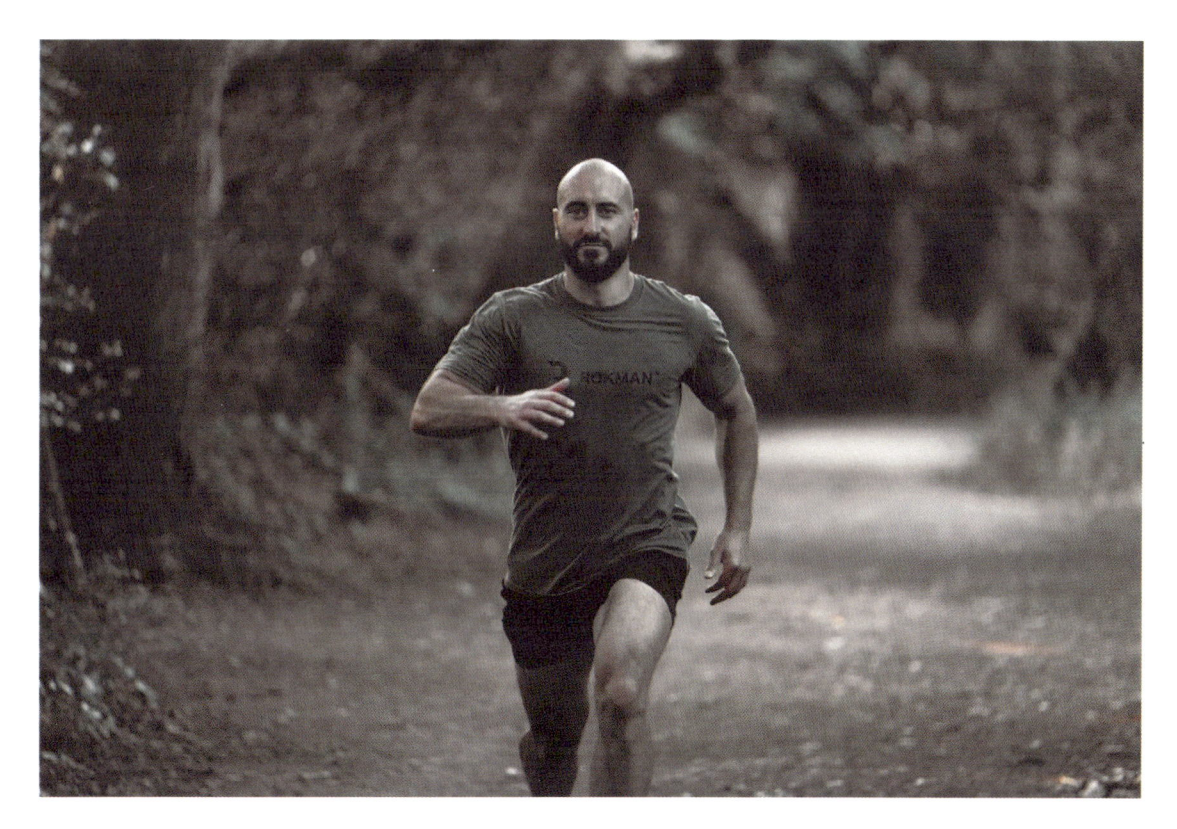

RUNNER

Max Glover

Above image and cover image credit: Rokman

Disclaimer:

1. Max Glover strongly recommends that you consult with your physician before beginning any exercise program. You should be in good physical condition and be able to participate in the exercise. Max Glover is not a licensed medical care provider and has no expertise in diagnosing, examining, or treating medical conditions of any kind, or in determining the effect of any specific exercise on a medical condition.
2. You should understand that when participating in any exercise or exercise program, there is the possibility of physical injury. If you engage in this exercise or exercise program, you agree that you do so at your own risk, are voluntarily participating in these activities, assume all risk of injury to yourself.
3. The information provided is not intended to be a substitute for professional medical advice, diagnosis or treatment. Never disregard professional medical advice, or delay in seeking it.
4. You are encouraged to consult with your doctor with regard to the information contained within this book.
5. Each individual's health, fitness, and nutrition success depends on his or her background, dedication, desire, and motivation. As with any health-related program or service, your results may vary, and will be based on many variables, including but not limited to, your individual capacity, life experience, unique health and genetic profile, starting point, expertise, and level of commitment.

Contents

- Introduction 7
- The Enjoyment of Running 8
- What is the 1.5 Mile Run Test? 9
- 1.5 Mile Run Minimum Standards 9
- Targets and goals 11
- Commando Nutrition 12
- Carbohydrates 13
- Proteins 13
- Fats 14
- Supplements 14
- Rest 15
- Rest During a Workout 15
- Rest Days (and when not exercising) 15
- Sleep 16
- Sleep Deprivation 16
- Commando: Runner 18
- Warm Up 18
- Hydration 19
- Safety 19
- Injuries / Feeling Unwell 19
- Muscle Activation 25
- Circuit Training 26
- Hill Sprints 27
- Steady Pace Runs 27
- Mobility and Dynamic Stretches 28
- Warm Up Exercises 31
- Exercises 33
- Stretches 38
- Testing 42
- Cadet Training Programme Schedule 44
- Day 1: 2 Mile Run 45
- Day 2: Walk 45
- Day 3: 2 Mile Run + Strength 46
- Day 4: Walk 46
- Day 5: 2 Mile Run 47

Day 6: Strength..47
Day 7: Rest..48
Day 8: 2.5 Mile Run...48
Day 9: Walk...49
Day 10: 2.5 Mile Run + Strength...49
Day 11: Walk...50
Day 12: 2.5 Mile Run...50
Day 13: Strength..51
Day 14: Rest..51
Day 15: 3 Mile Run..52
Day 16: Walk...52
Day 17: 3 Mile Run + Strength..53
Day 18: Walk...53
Day 19: 3 Mile Run..54
Day 20: Strength..54
Day 21: Rest..55
Day 22: 3.5 Mile Run...55
Day 23: Walk...56
Day 24: 3.5 Mile Run + Strength...56
Day 25: Walk...57
Day 26: 3.5 Mile Run...57
Day 27: Strength..58
Day 28: Rest..58
Day 29: 4 Mile Run..59
Day 30: Walk...59
Day 31: 4 Mile Run + Strength..60
Day 32: Walk...60
Day 33: 4 Mile Run..61
Day 34: Strength..62
Day 35: Rest..62
Day 36: 4.5 Mile Run...63
Day 37: Walk...63
Day 38: 4.5 Mile Run + Strength...64
Day 39: Walk...64
Day 40: 4.5 Mile Run...65
Day 41: Strength..65

Day 42: Rest 66
Test Week Schedule 66
Day 1: Rest 66
Day 2: Test 67
Day 3: Walk 67
Day 4: 3 Mile Run + Strength 68
Day 5: Walk 68
Day 6: Strength 69
Day 7: Rest 69
Recruit Training Programme Schedule 70
Day 1: 5 Mile Run 71
Day 2: Walk 71
Day 3: Hill Sprints + Strength 72
Day 4: Walk 72
Day 5: 4 Mile Run 73
Day 6: Strength 73
Day 7: Rest 74
Day 8: 5.5 Mile Run 74
Day 9: Walk 75
Day 10: Hill Sprints + Strength 75
Day 11: Walk 76
Day 12: 4 Mile Run 76
Day 13: Strength 77
Day 14: Rest 77
Day 15: 6 Mile Run 78
Day 16: Walk 78
Day 17: Hill Sprints + Strength 79
Day 18: Walk 79
Day 19: 4 Mile Run 80
Day 20: Strength 80
Day 21: Rest 81
Day 22: 6.5 Mile Run 81
Day 23: Walk 82
Day 24: Hill Sprints + Strength 82
Day 25: Walk 83
Day 26: 800m Sprints 83

Day 27: Strength..84
Day 28: Rest..84
Day 29: 7 Mile Run 85
Day 30: Walk...85
Day 31: Hill Sprints + Strength..86
Day 32: Walk...86
Day 33: 800 Metre Sprints..87
Day 34: Strength..88
Day 35: Rest...88
Day 36: 7.5 Mile Run 89
Day 37: Walk...89
Day 38: Hill Sprints + Strength..90
Day 39: Walk...90
Day 40: 800 metre sprints 91
Day 41: Strength..92
Day 42: Rest...92
Day 43: Rest...93
Day 44: Test 94
Beyond Commando Runner 94
Alternative Exercises..97
Author Profile 99

Introduction

Welcome to the Commando Runner training programme. The aim of this programme is to make you run stronger, faster and increase your fitness and endurance. While it has a military theme, civilian runners can benefit greatly as well.

This course is ideal for:

- Individuals seeking to get fit to join the military
- Serving military personnel who wish to gain an edge over their peers
- Police and law enforcement
- Runners who are training for races such as 5k, 10k and half marathons

Please read the supporting information and then make your way through the training plan. It is designed for you to fill in as you go, it details what to do on each day of the programme and doubles up as a training log. (It is suggested for those purchasing the eBook version on Kindle that they should use the notes function within the app to record their training data).

To track performance progress the programme uses the 1.5 mile run test. After the initial test, individuals have three routes to take:

1. Developmental Running Programme
2. Cadet Programme (Foundation Phase)
3. Recruit Training Programme

Each phase ends with a fitness test to track your progress.

More Than Just a Running Programme

Commandos are not only excellent runners; they are also strong and mentally robust. The aim of this programme is to enhance physical fitness, mental resilience, wellbeing and give you the tools to continue improving even after the course has ended. As you become better at running, it becomes a very enjoyable experience.

Please take your time to familiarise yourself with the accompanying information before starting, and then work your way through the guide whilst giving 100%.

I'd like to thank you for purchasing a copy of Commando Runner and I wish you the very best and success in your goals.

The Enjoyment of Running

As a young Bootneck, very few things excited me more than going out for a fast, hard run. At the peak of my physical fitness, we would run up hills and mountains. At the top I would admire the view and breathe in the fresh air. When people refer to "the runners high" this is what I think of.

I was quite lucky. During my service in the Royal Marines, I spent a lot of my time training in the mountains of Scotland. We would regularly run up long and steep mountain roads. What would start off a slow paced jog to warm up in the cold winter mornings would soon turn into a competitive race up the hills, some of which were over a mile long slog.

We wore the Green Beret and we were not only united by our headdress, but also by our desire to push ourselves harder. I remember each training session fondly. Intense running sessions every other morning. Spontaneous 10 milers for fun, fireman's carry races up the steepest hill we could find, hill sprints and every recruit's favourite - it pays to be a winner.

The result was, we possessed a seemingly limitless ability to run.

As a new Commando; I distinctly remember returning home and running with some civilian friends and leaving them in the dust without even realising it. I briefly joined a rugby team and while I had no skill, I ran rings around the other players. Running soon became my preferred method of travel, I'd even gladly crack the 5 mile run home from a night out in town to save money on the taxi fare!

The fitness standards for Royal Marines are high and for a good reason. After the run, speed march or yomp they are expected to be ready to fight.

If you imagine running a race, such as a 10k, half marathon or obstacle course race. At the end you'd probably want to have a sit down, recover and relax. From a Royal Marines perspective, when you reach that part – the hard stuff is just about to begin.

We had to be fit because we were expected to perform at our best when we were tired. Our performance at the job could have been the difference between life and death. The stakes were high. We trained so hard that running on any terrain over any distance and pace became enjoyable for us.

I want this training manual to be a bridge from me to you, sharing my knowledge from what I experienced in the Marines but also in subsequent years of training and study.

If you read this programme, you will have significantly more training knowledge than I had as an 18 year old when I went through recruit training to earn my green beret. I hope that you can make use of this knowledge and whether you're training to join the Marines or not, I hope that it can help you experience the enjoyment of running and being fit.

What is the 1.5 Mile Run Test?

The 1.5 Mile (2.4km) Run is a simple test method employed by many military units such as the British Special Forces and US Navy SEALs to quickly assess a soldier's fitness. It is easy to perform and can be done virtually anywhere. What makes it useful for the military is that a large number of candidates can perform the test in a short amount of time as all that is required is a running surface and a stopwatch. The relatively short distance of this test means it is too long for a full-on sprint but also too short for a slow-paced effort.

This is why many people struggle and fail to reach their potential on this test. They simply do not develop the systems to be able to push themselves for the 8-10 minutes required.

Many different Military Units use similar distances (US Marines use a 3-mile run, and others use a 1.86m run). This training programme will use the 1.5 mile run test a standardised testing method.

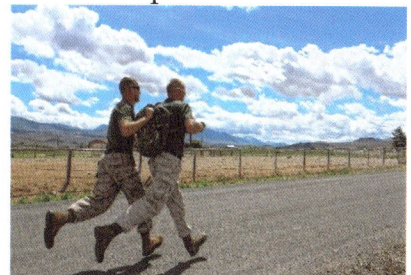

1.5 Mile Run Minimum Standards

For interest purposes, see below table for the various different countries armies and military units that use the 1.5 mile run test. Listed are the minimum required standards for a male candidate. Some test will allow different pass scores for age and gender.

Usually, the running test will accompany other tests such as press ups, pull ups, shuttle runs, fireman's carries etc. The listed minimums do not guarantee a pass or entry into the military but will add to the candidate's overall score. Candidates are often encouraged to seek higher scores on these tests.

Military Unit / Regiment	Minimum 1.5 Mile Run Time
Australian Defence Force	11:18 – 15:30 (age dependent)
British Army*	12:40
Irish Army	11:40
Luxembourg Army	14:30
New Zealand Army	10:30
Royal Marines*	10:30
South African Defence Force	12:00
UK Parachute Regiment*	9:40
UK Special Air Service	09:30
US Air Force	13:13 – 18:14 (age dependent)
US Coast Guard	12:51
US Navy SEALs	10:30

Fitness tests have recently been changed, but have been included for interest purposes.

Note – I cannot guarantee the accuracy of these fitness test scores as they can change and many armed forces do not openly share their fitness test information. If you are in the joining process for any of these military units, please confirm the fitness test requirements with your recruiter.

How Fit Are Royal Marines Commandos?

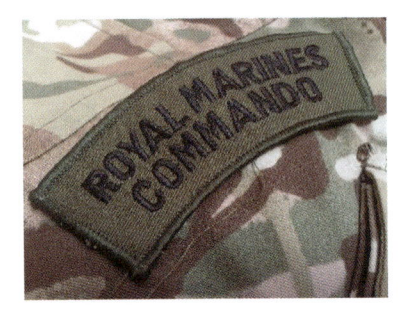

Being 100% straight with you… Soldiers from elite military regiments do not struggle to reach the minimum criteria for this test. In fact, when I served in the Royal Marines, we had to do this test twice a year and it was a joke to us. We would do it for fun. It was not unheard of for Royal Marines Commandos to complete the 1.5 mile run in sub 8 minutes every time, without training specifically for this test.

Royal Marines training is tough and the fitness element is a mixture of running, circuit training, assault courses and loaded marches. Their fitness programme is designed to prepare them for the rigours and demands of combat.

I am going to share with you some of the training techniques that I used as a young Marine and also as a civilian to get fitter and faster.

The techniques listed in this programme work. After I had left the Marines, I had a very unhealthy period of my life where I drank and smoked way too much. I decided to ditch the crap and train for a half marathon (13.1 miles). After only 3 months of training, I ran the half marathon in 1:25. This was at a bodyweight of 91kg and was still able to perform 12 solid pull ups and bench press 130kg. Commandos not only need to be fit, but they need to be strong too.

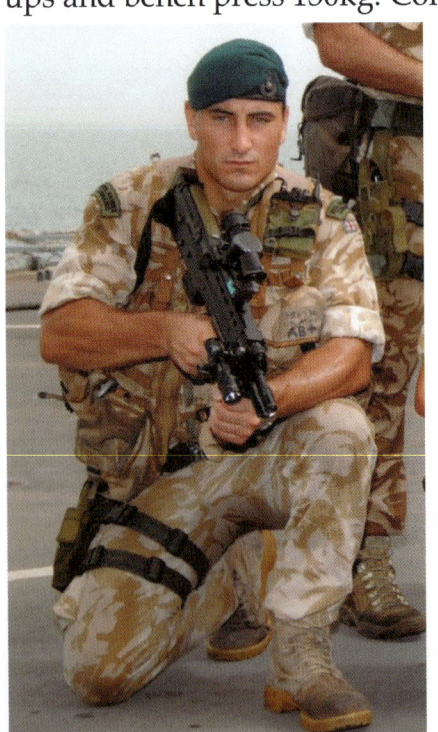

In 2015, having not ran at all for 6 years I applied to join the British Army and scored a sub-9-minute 1.5 mile run time during the selection, with only 2 weeks of training.

My personal record on the 20-metre bleep test was level 16 and I wasn't doing any long distance running at the time.

The purpose of this training programme is to:

- Ascertain your current fitness and highlight any weaknesses
- Build up stamina
- Increase psychological focus

I studied my successes and many failures over the years; before I joined the Marines, during my service and also the years that followed. Everything included in this programme is there for a purpose.

Targets and goals

Here's your first assignment. Write down your target goal – you are 42% more likely to achieve your goal if you write them down. This programme contains a daily training log for you to complete. Record your achievements and set yourself goals and challenges. Don't pay lip service this, it is important.

Mind set and motivation – sometimes it will be hard to motivate yourself to go and train. Break your longer runs down in your head.

1. Put your trainers on
2. Get outside
3. Get that first mile done

You can do those three things and by the time you have done 1 mile you will be kicking ass.

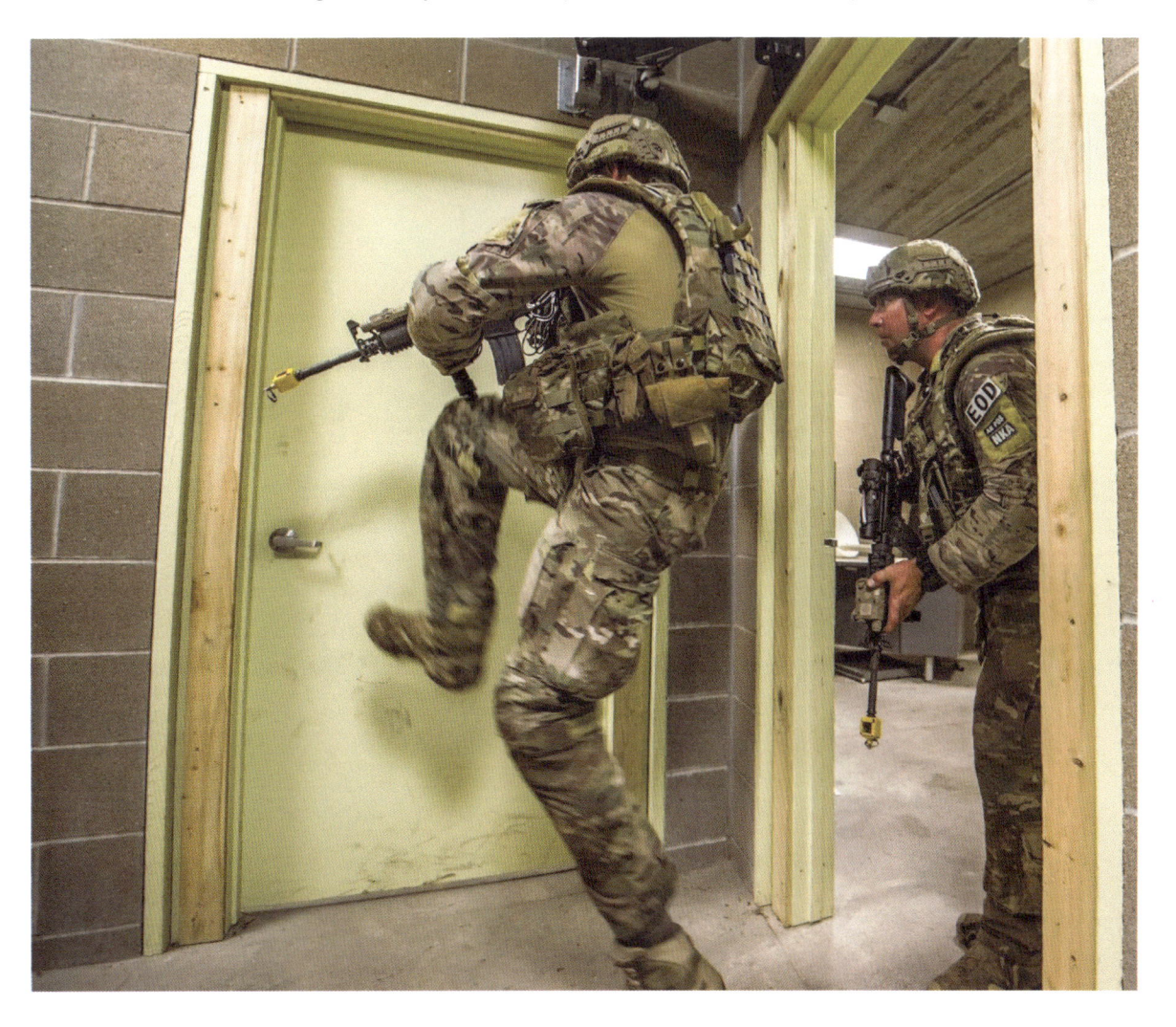

Commando Runner does not just contain running. It consists of a variety of different training methods to help you achieve your goal:

> Steady state long runs
> Moderate intensity runs
> Hill sprints
> Long sprints
> Strength training
> Bodyweight circuits

Commando Nutrition

What you put in your body can enhance your success. Consuming good quality and nutritious foods will boost your health and your performance. I have included some basic nutrition information that should be useful to you achieving your goals.

Don't forget that nutritious food doesn't have to be boring.

It is important that you plan your nutrition. Ensure that you always have adequate food to support your training. Remember that food is your fuel!

Asking yourself these questions can help you on the path to results:

- Are you eating enough before your run?
    - When training for performance, having the fuel in your system can make a huge difference
    - Carbohydrates are the most efficient fuel source – they are broken down by your body into glucose and either used immediately or stored in your muscles as glycogen
    - When you are running your body will use the glucose that it has immediately available. During intense exercise this will quickly run out and then your body will use its glycogen stores
- Are you eating enough protein?
    - When you run, your muscle tissue breaks down, consuming protein will help your muscles rebuild after exercise
- Are you avoiding fat?
    - Fat is a backup fuel, particularly when running longer distances
    - Some fats are healthy and packed with nutrients, others like trans fats found in fried foods, margarine and hydrogenated oils are unhealthy, should be avoided and give the other types of fat a bad rep
    - Healthy fats can help reduce inflammation and athletes who consume sufficient healthy fats may be able to recover better from training

Remember – that eating healthy, fresh food containing a variety of vitamins and minerals will help not only improve your performance during your workout, but will likely enhance your recovery. This will promote continued performance and results in the long term.

Carbohydrates

Carbs are the body's primary energy source. Good quality carbohydrates can fuel your training and increase performance.

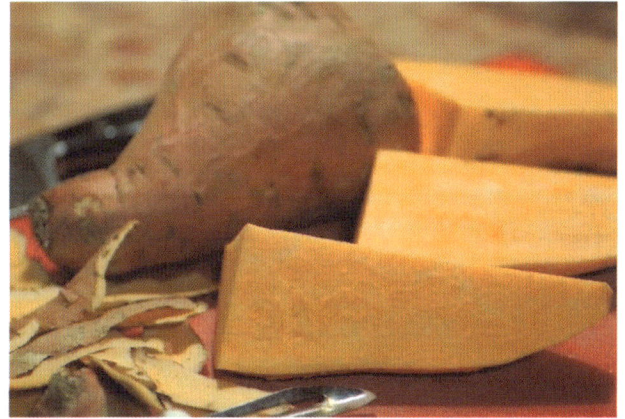

Complex carbs such as:
- Oats
- Bread
- Sweet potatoes
- Yams
- Brown rice
- Wholewheat pasta

Fruits such as bananas and berries are good sources of quick carbohydrates, that could be used as pre or post workout, however for your main meals try and stick to the complex carbs.

Adding nutrient dense foods such as beetroot to your plate can be really useful and could also provide your workouts with a powerful boost.

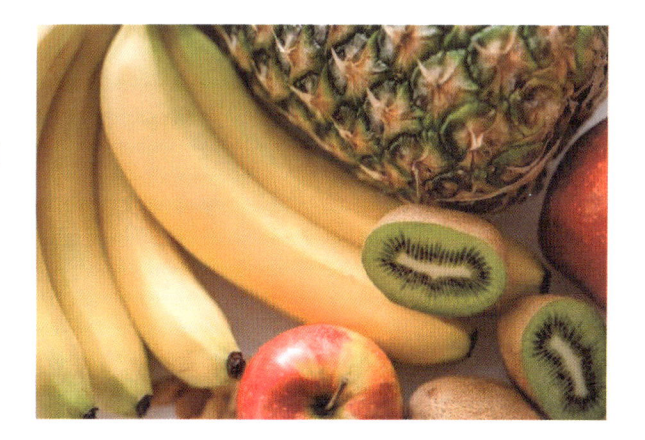

An ideal amount for this programme is 7-10 grams of carbs per kg of bodyweight.

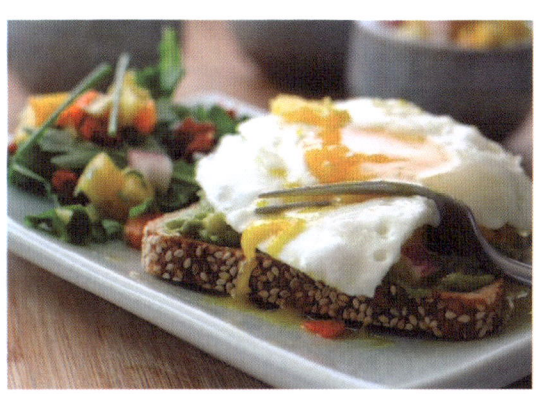

Proteins

Examples:
- Eggs
- Fish
- Chicken
- Red meat (try and go for the leanest meat)

As a general rule try and limit the amount of processed meat you consume.
Aim to consume 1.2-2 grams of protein per kg of bodyweight.

Fats

- Avocados
- Nuts and seeds
- Oily fish such as sardines

20-30% of daily calories should come from fat.

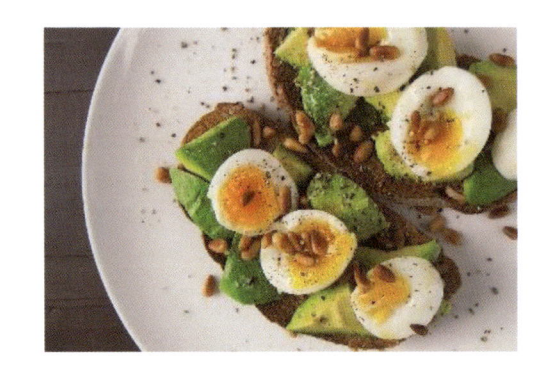

Dietary fats are not quickly converted by your body into fuel, but they are essential for helping your body absorb vitamins.

Supplements

Caffeine – Can offer a pre-workout boost (no need to take any fancy powders, a cup of coffee should suffice). If you are consuming caffeine, be aware that it can stay active in your system for a few hours and could potentially affect your sleep.

Creatine – Can allow some people to perform better at shorter fast sessions such as sprints. Optimum dosage would be at 5g per day, post workout.

Whey protein – to assist with muscle repair following intense training sessions.

Magnesium – Assists with nerve function, energy and muscle contractions. Optimum time to take this very important mineral as a supplement would be before bed as it may help you relax and sleep better, assisting with enhanced recovery.

Green Tea – Drinking green tea may help with fat oxidation, which could increase endurance and performance levels.

Supplements cannot replace a complete, healthy balanced diet. So before even considering taking any supplements make sure that you have your nutrition in check.

<u>**Are Supplements Essential?**</u>

No, they are not essential. A Complete and balanced diet is the most important thing. I did not take supplements whilst I was training for the Marines, nor during recruit training – yet I was successful. The supplements I have listed above are ones that I have used in the years after and I found them to be of benefit.

Rest

Why is rest important? When you train, your body responds in the period of time after training to adapt and get fitter. If you trained hard every single day, partied every night surviving on less than 2 hours sleep only to repeat this process every single day for a year what sort of state do you think you would be in?

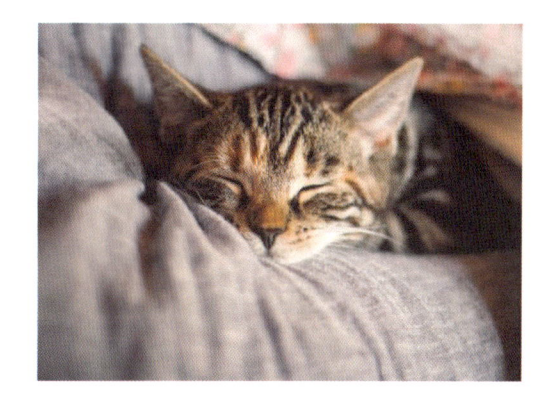

Rest falls into a few categories:

Rest During a Workout

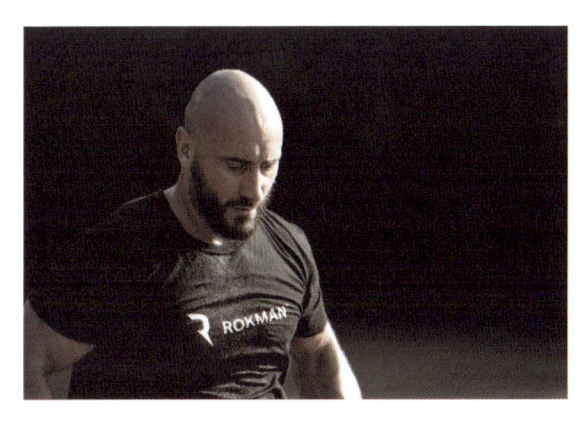

This is the period where you take breaks during your exercise. The harder and more intense the exercise is the more rest period you would likely require. For example, when doing a set of hill sprints, you would not be sprinting continuously during the session. It would be more effective to work hard for a short period of time followed by a rest period that is just long enough for you to be able to try and repeat that same intense effort.

As you get fitter, the less rest period you will require. Someone who is unfit, new to training or recovering from an injury will require a longer rest period. In those circumstances, short rest periods could also be needed for moderate or even low intensity exercises.

Rest Days (and when not exercising)

Rest days (or the remainder of the training day) does not mean lying in bed all day doing nothing. Ideally try and limit the amount of stress you put on your body. You will likely not be able to recover as quickly from an intense training session if you're also spending another few hours playing sports or some other intense activity.

However, performing light forms of exercise such as walking or stretching will be beneficial and could assist recovery and improve your physical and mental wellbeing. It is for this reason that I have included them in the Commando Runner programme. I am not saying do not participate in any sports, however I would suggest adjusting your programme to accommodate for the sport in such a way that neither your running training or your extra-curricular activity does not suffer as a consequence.

A lot of this does come down to prioritising your goals. Many of us would love to be able to participate in several sports at a high level, build muscle, lose bodyfat, lift the big boy weights, run marathons and sprint the 100m like Usain Bolt. However, we simply cannot be a master of all trades. Especially when we consider things like work, family, children, hobbies and other commitments we may have.

Sleep

Sleep is a very important function of the body. It allows the brain and body to recharge, keeps the body and mind healthy and functioning correctly. Regular poor sleep can increase your chances of obesity, heart disease and diabetes. Health experts also warn that it can shorten your life expectancy. This shows that sleep is absolutely fundamental in allowing our bodies to function and perform at an optimum level.

Remember
Consistent lack of sleep can lower your testosterone levels, reduce your immune system and obliterate your sex drive.

Sleep Deprivation

If you have ever been a shift worker or served in the military you will know a thing or two about sleep deprivation. However, many individuals from these backgrounds believe they do not need to sleep 8 hours per night to function. They state that they are used to it, and well… they are part right.

The human body is absolutely amazing at adapting to whatever is thrown at it. So, in the case of the shift worker who operates on a handful of hours sleep here and there, they are actually in a perpetual state of tiredness. The only thing is – their bodies have got used to feeling tired and so feeling tired becomes normal.

Can you remember a time 2 years ago and remember how tired or awake you were feeling on a given day and compare it with how tired you are today? Unlikely. Can you compare how tired or awake you felt yesterday and compare it with how tired today? Quite possibly.

An individual who consistently gets less than 6 hours sleep can suffer the same drop in performance over a period of 2 weeks as an individual who sleeps 8 hours a week suffers by staying awake for over 24 hours. The difference is the person getting 8 hours sleep notices it and feels like trash. Whereas the person who is consistently sleep deprived does not notice it due to the gradual decline and the "re-norming" process, and in turn does not recognise their drop in performance.

So yes, we can get used to not sleeping, however the health consequences will be building up underneath the surface.

If you need further convincing what this also means is if you don't get enough quality sleep:

> 1. **Your running will not improve to its full potential**
> 2. **Your testosterone will dramatically decrease – even if you are young and healthy (it's worse for anyone over 30 too!)**
> 3. **You're more likely to get injured and be sick**

I believe sleep is so paramount to performance I have included a sleep diary within this programme that I strongly advise you to make use of.

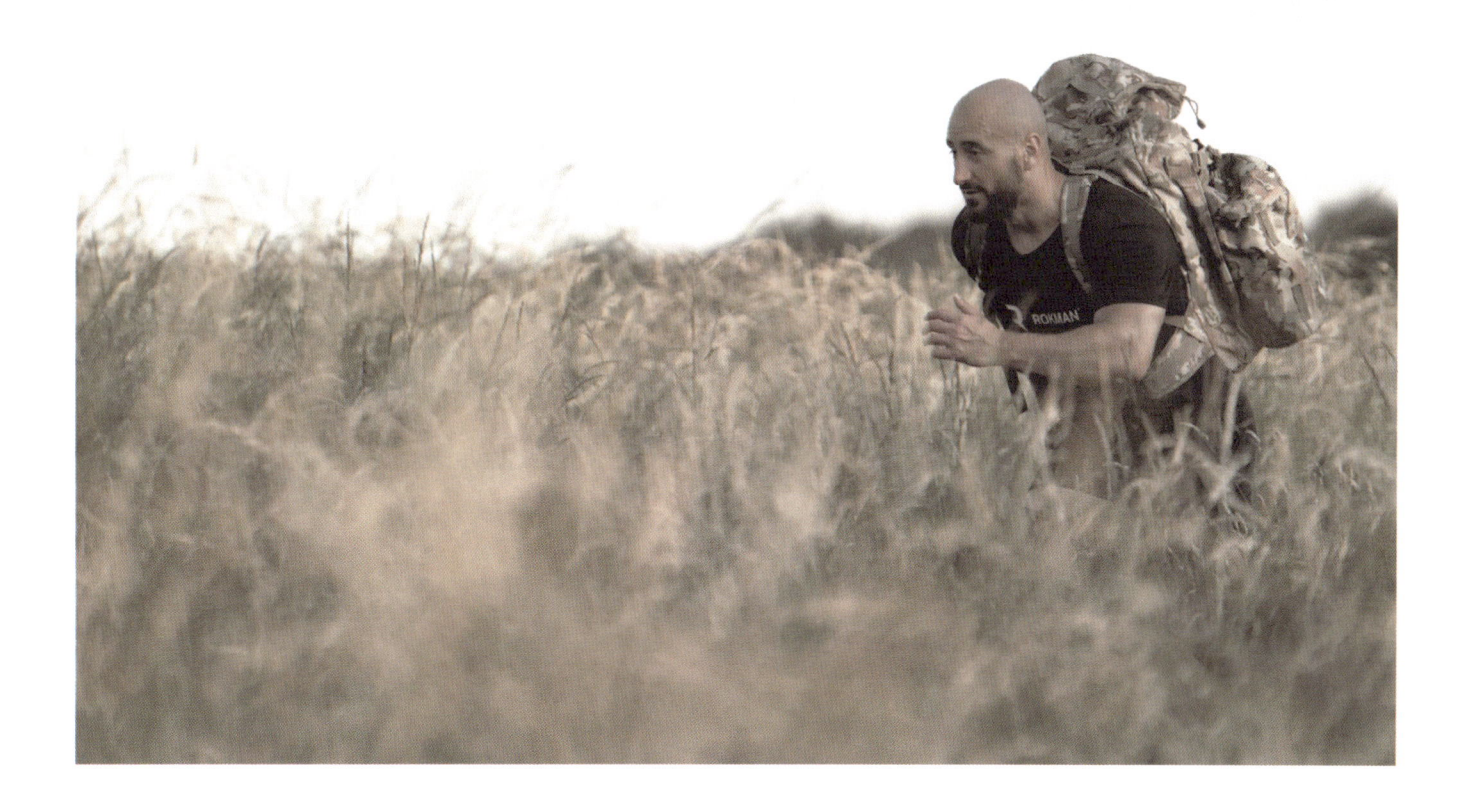

Commando: Runner

Please read the programme details carefully, and pay attention to the supporting information.

If you have any injuries or medical conditions that could be negatively affected by intense exercise, please do not begin this programme.

You are responsible for ensuring that you are exercising in a safe environment, and make sure you wear appropriate exercise attire suitable to the conditions throughout.

To be Successful follow these rules...

Warm Up

All workouts must begin with a thorough warm up. Remember the acronym **RAMP**, and follow this procedure:

Raise blood flow, muscle temperature, core temperature, muscle elasticity through low intensity movements
Activate & Mobilise Your muscles and joints with dynamic movements
Potentiate The movements you are doing in the workout, e.g., gradually increase the weight you are doing on a squat, or build up speed on short sprints

Warming up correctly can not only reduce the likelihood of injury but can improve performance. Warm ups should be specific to the workout.

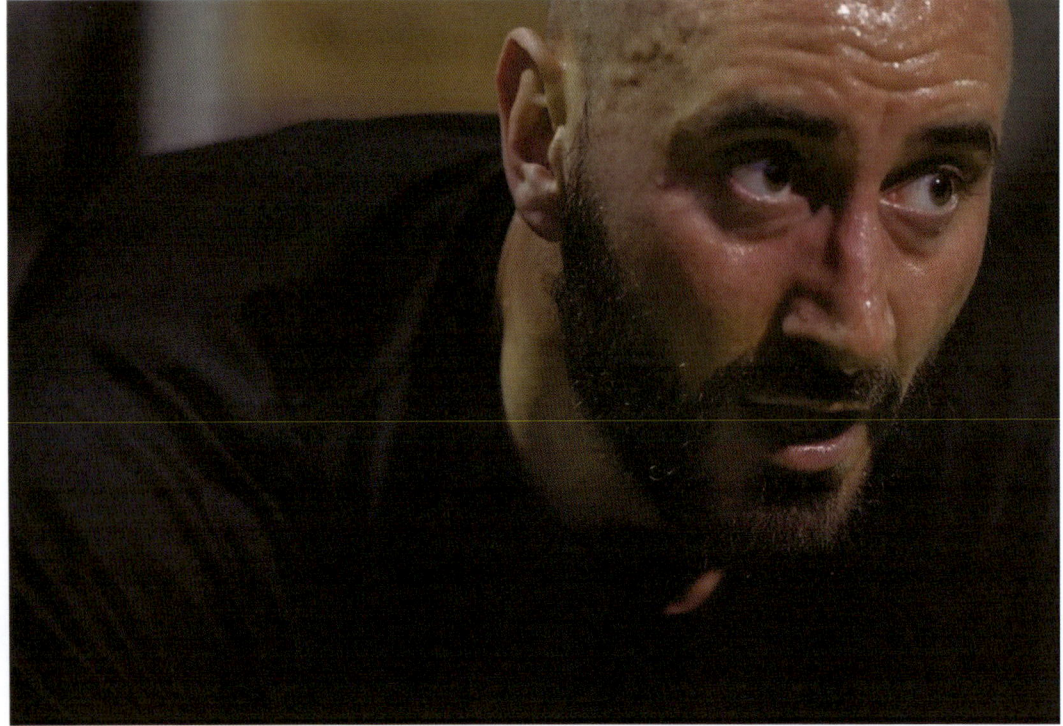

Hydration

It is imperative that you stay hydrated throughout the day by drinking plenty of water. The easiest way to stay on top of this is to check the colour of your urine. Ideally it should be clear or a pale yellow. If it's dark yellow you need to drink more water. Make sure that you have drinking water with you during your runs, walks and circuit training sessions.

Safety

You are responsible for your route selection, it is advisable to select a route that is adequately lit, with good firm flooring and does not involve you going out on the road. You should wear high visibility clothing and appropriate training attire at all times. When going on a run / sprint you should make others aware that you are going out, what you are doing, where you are going and an estimated time of return.

Injuries / Feeling Unwell

Pushing through a workout when you're injured or unwell is not smart and injuries are not a badge of honour. If at any point you feel unwell or become injured during this training programme you must stop immediately, contact your doctor and not resume the programme until you have had permission from a medical professional. If you do need to stop or take additional breaks from this programme that is fine, there are scheduled rests in the programme but everyone is different and some people take longer to recover than others. You can insert additional rests in as you see fit and just carry the programme on from there.

This train line represents your journey through the programme:

If you get injured for whatever reason you must stop, it is simply like getting off at a stop and waiting for your next train to continue your journey.

Once you are ready to continue your journey then it is a good idea to start off a little bit further behind as you will have lost some of your gains and this will give you the opportunity to build back up.

It's very important to accept this process. Many a trainee has fallen victim to not allowing their body to heal for being concerned about not achieving their fitness goals. The longer and harder you train on an injury the longer it will take to recover. You will not be able to perform at your potential if you are limping around in pain. **Stop, rest, recover, rehabilitate and get going again.**

What's also equally important and often overlooked is reflection. And I'm not talking about checking yourself out in the mirror. If you develop an injury then it is a wise idea to try and understand how this happened. What led to this happening? If the injury is a result of direct blunt trauma (such as a sports injury) it doesn't take a detective to figure out the cause, but don't always take the apparent reason at face value.

A lot of injuries occur due to a build-up in poor training practices, tight, weak or unbalanced muscles. These injuries may sometimes manifest themselves by doing something seemingly harmless like picking up an object from the floor or putting on the trousers.

Once you identify how and why the injury occurred then use this as an opportunity to put steps in place to prevent it from happening again.

I learnt the hard way. One Summer many years ago I decided I didn't want to skip a gym session that I was not ready for. Having partied until the early hours of the morning celebrating my friend's birthday - drinking copious amounts of alcohol and getting next to no sleep I went straight into a long shift at work.

At the time I was a door supervisor and was doing security for a very busy event. Much to my annoyance the air conditioning had packed in on one of the hottest days of the year. Dressed in a suit I was sweating my bollocks off fighting with intoxicated punters.

When I got home that night, I noticed I was suffering mild symptoms of heat illness. Not a problem at the time – I was trained to recognise it and dealt with it, then I went to bed. The next day was my day off. I knew I wasn't 100% but decided to hit the gym for what was scheduled to be an intense squat session. In my head I proposed that I would just do a light workout and continue my schedule in a couple of days. Fate however, had other arrangements for me.

Upon arrival at the gym, I was filling up my water bottle at the fountain when the hottest girl in the gym appeared out of nowhere and decided to engage me in conversation. The macho man in me quickly quelled the idea of performing a light weight workout… I didn't want to look like a pussy so I marched over to continue my heavy session – neglecting my warm up.

During my second set of squats, I gripped the bar, took a deep breath lowered myself down and as I was about to push up felt an intense explosion in the back of my head. My vision blurred and an intense pain that was worse than any kick or punch to the head I have ever experienced. (And I've taken a few!)

Being me, I continued my workout, and subsequent sessions after that for 2 weeks. However, during these 2 weeks I experienced blinding headaches, memory loss and slurring of words.

Eventually I gave in and went to see a Doctor, I had sustained a brain injury and had to take 6 months off training or any physical activity that could raise my blood pressure. Upon returning to the gym my muscles had become weak and I ended up pulling my adductor, which set me back even further.

So, the outcome of this story is:

1. Rather than skipping one session I forfeited over 6 months!
2. I let my ego get the better of me which probably made the damage even worse

What I learnt from this:

1. I never skip a warm up – if anything I warm up too much now
2. I will only train when I am ready to train
3. I stopped drinking alcohol (apart from the odd special occasion)

Performance Mindset

I left the Royal Marines and pretty much stopped running all together. Six years later, I applied to join the British Army. During my initial interview I spoke with the recruitment Sergeant who asked me how much running I was doing.

"I haven't run for years," I told him.

He told me that I had better start doing some running and asked me what time I would expect on the 1.5 mile run during the aptitude tests.

"Under 9 minutes," was my response.

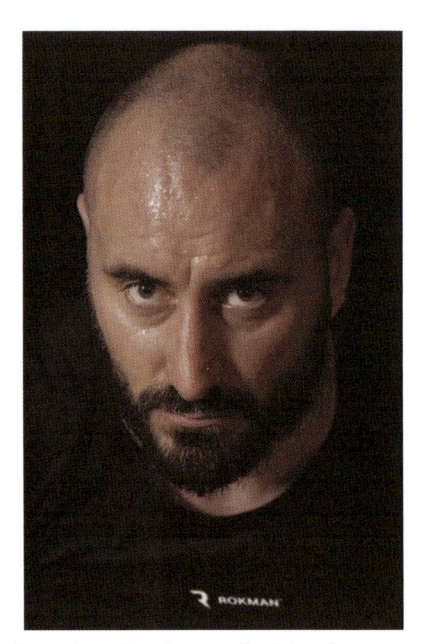

The Sergeant laughed and advised me that I didn't need a time that fast for the branch I had applied for and proceeded with the interview. There had been some concerns due to my weight and lack of running however, the Sergeant was a good bloke and gave me the benefit of the doubt, approving me to attend the next selection course.

I performed 6 training runs over the next 2 weeks and attended the selection course as the oldest and heaviest candidate. The 1.5 mile run was the first test and after a 200 metre warm up walk, followed by 30 seconds of stretches; we were off. We ran laps of the small Army base until we hit the distance of 1.5 miles and I achieved a time of 8 minutes 59 seconds, the second fastest time on the course.

How had I gone from a non-runner to keeping up with and beating younger people who had been training for months, even years during a selection test for a career that they really wanted, yet one that I wasn't particularly that bothered about?

The answer is in the **performance mindset**.

While physical training is crucial to your success, an often-overlooked aspect of a fitness programme is mindset. If you have got a weak mind, or are simply not in the right frame of mind throughout, it is unlikely you will be able to perform to your full potential.

You will often hear people state that they are "bringing their A-Game", "Getting in the zone" or "putting their war face on"

These are sayings that depict the mental transition someone is taking to allow them to perform at their best. Here are some mindset approaches that can be used to increase your performance in fitness, sport, work or life in general.

Focus

Divert your attention to one thing and be disciplined about it (in this case it is improving your run time). Focus your mind on solely thinking about improving your running - hitting that sub 9 1.5 mile run time (or whatever your aim is).

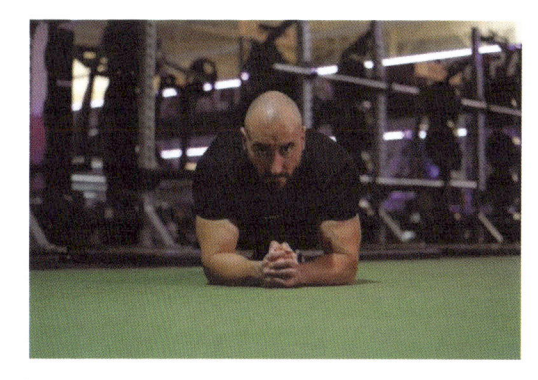

When I had fitness a goal, I was thinking about them so hard I was even dreaming about them. When I wanted to be a better runner, I'd be running for training when I wasn't training, I was thinking about running. As a passenger in a vehicle, I would look out of the window at the countryside passing by and imagine that I was running through the fields and woodlands at the same speed as the car. When I was trying to build my muscles, I was doing bench presses in my sleep – much to the annoyance of anyone who shared a bed with me!

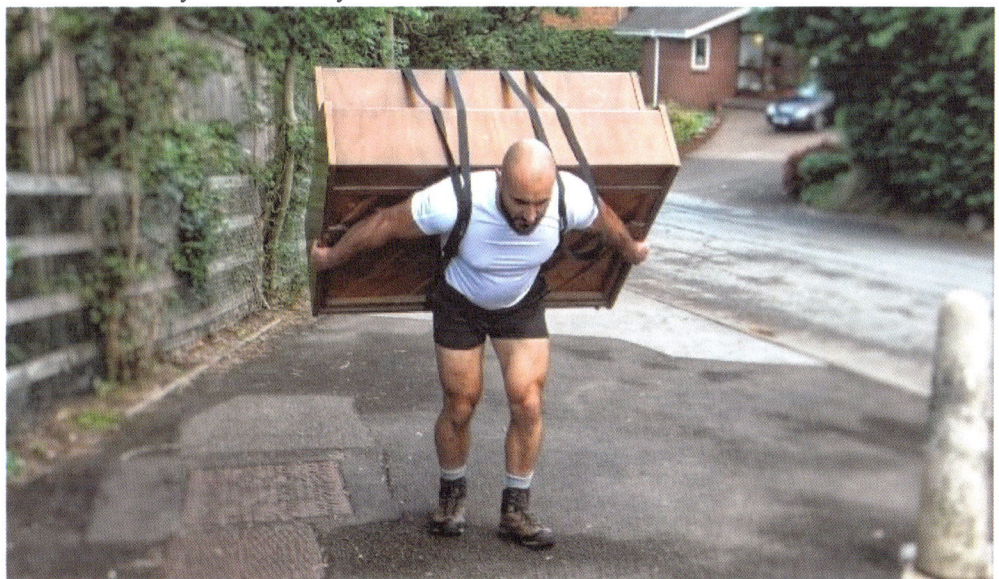

If you're easily distracted or sitting their playing on your phone all evening and not thinking about your goals then you will be lacking the focus to move onto the next step.

Visualisation - imaging doing it. Achieving it. Think it over and over and over in your head become obsessed with it. When I was training to carry a piano up a mountain - it wasn't new for me when I got to the top because I'd already been there. I'd walked the whole route in my head with an imaginary piano on my back. I knew the steps I had to take. I prepared so well for this challenge that once I got going on the day of the event, it was relatively easy for me.

Make a Start – some days you feel lazy and rubbish. It's a fact, I don't care who you are, every single one of us has days where we just cannot be bothered to train. I have been there on countless occasions. THESE ARE THE DAYS THAT COUNT. If you feel this way just get up put your trainers on and make a start, commit to doing just a warm up, mobility session, short walk or gentle jog…. Then once the blood is flowing that focus will return. (I will add a note to this, if you are completely overworked, ill or injured this rule may not apply, then it is best to rest and recuperate. You will have to be the judge of that).

Recognise Your Achievements – we all like to win. Knocking 1 second off your time is a victory so celebrate it. Multiple wins will set you on a roll to success.

Remember Why You Are Doing This – This is a powerful tool to have in your arsenal. It can link in heavily with the visualisation principle as mentioned earlier. When I was working shifts and training towards a bodybuilding goal, I remember sitting on the bench press tired, flat, unmotivated and the weight feeling heavy. In my head I would visualise my goal – the end product and think about why I was doing this, I'd move my arms, push them out to the front, swing them across my chest, tense the muscle – whatever to get the blood flowing through them, lie down and smash out a heavy set.

Marginal Gains –every single thing you do is one small step towards your goal. These incremental improvements may seem insignificant in isolation but when added together becomes a snowball effect. I call this the 100% Principle – of all the serious challenges I have attempted, trained and prepared for – the goal of completing this was assigned the value of 100% and all my efforts contributing towards the goal were assigned % value to take me towards that goal.

Step Out of Your Comfort Zone – this was the hardest thing for me to do in my younger days. I was so afraid of failure, afraid of looking stupid. Because I trained hard and was in good shape and had a bit of an ego, I was so concerned about what other people would think if I failed something that on some occasions I wouldn't even try if I suspected I wouldn't be very good at it. The point is… I never tried.

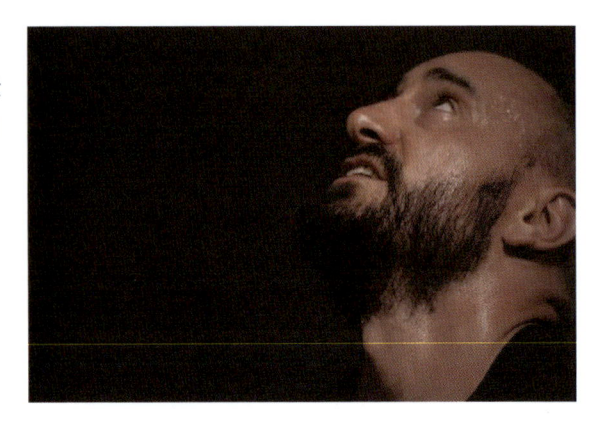

Enjoy the Journey – Our lives constantly change, what are goals now in years to come will be just memories. What you experience on your journey will have a more lasting impact on your character than the results.

Muscle Activation

Quite often when people think about running programmes all they think about is the running aspect of it. While of course, this is crucial but there often many things overlooked. One of these is muscle activation within the glutes, or lack of. Exercises like the side lying leg lifts and glute bridges may seem mundane and are included in most days of the programme they are incredibly important and not something that should be skipped.

If you imagine you are an engineer tasked with building a high-performance sports car. The manufacturer has given you a car and instructed you to maximise performance. Would you leave the car exactly how it is and hope that it somehow gets better? Or would you continuously try and tweak and upgrade the vehicle to get the best performance out of it?

That's exactly the same with your body. By regularly exercising the glutes we can awaken them and harness the power from these muscles. Modern life and sedentary sitting and general inactivity has caused our glutes to become lazy. These exercises will help give them that kick up the ass they need to engage correctly and take your performance to the next level. And just like laying a house brick by brick, doing these exercises regularly will build a solid foundation.

The glutes generate power and lots of it! They're also responsible for stabilising the pelvis. By activating these muscles to fire on all cylinders you are seriously upgrading your potential!

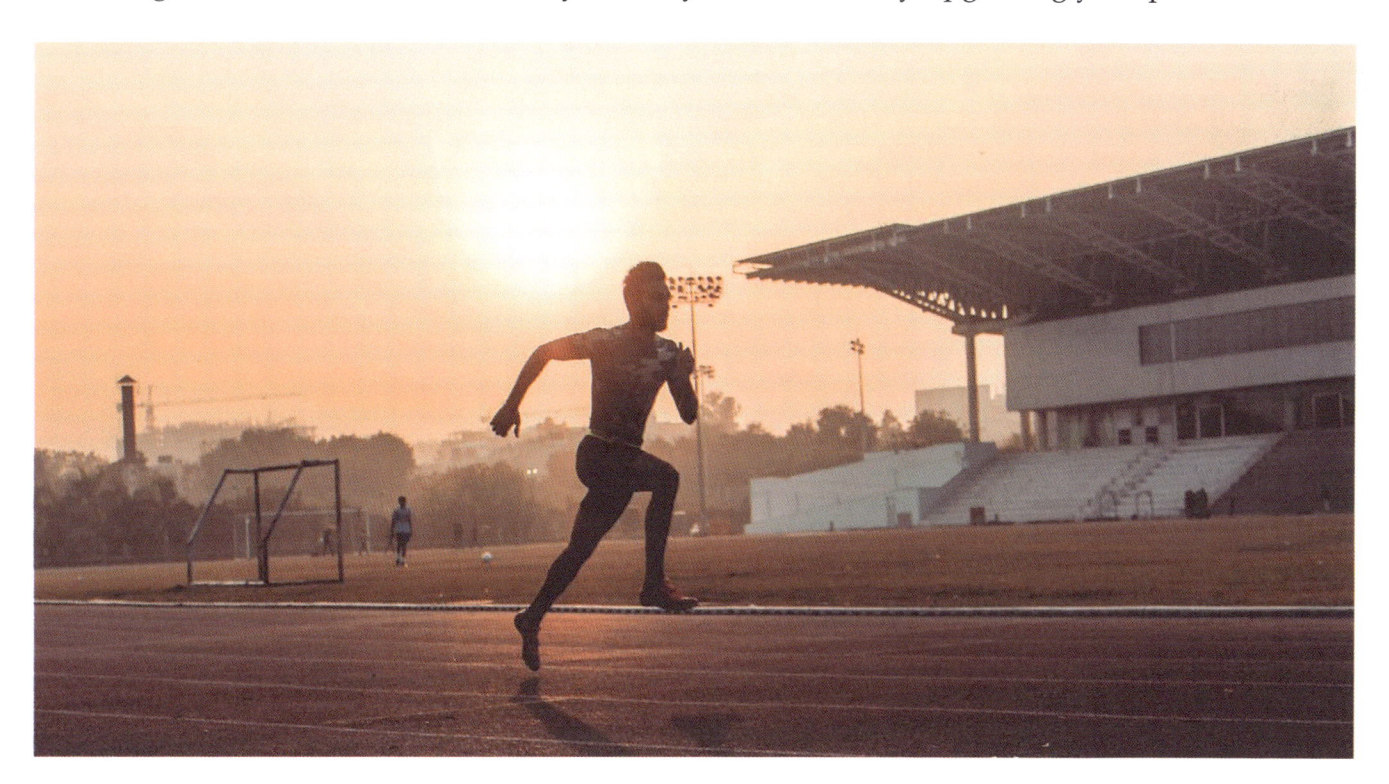

Circuit Training

The running in this programme is accompanied with a strength circuit. This begins with bodyweight only and will progress in number of repetitions and also in resistance. Some exercises can be progressed to include weights if required.

Set a stop watch to time your circuit, take minimal rest between each exercise. Ensure you are using good form to complete the exercises. Do not execute the exercises with bad form to improve your time. If your form breaks down during an exercise before you have completed the specified number of repetitions, rest and continue when you are ready.

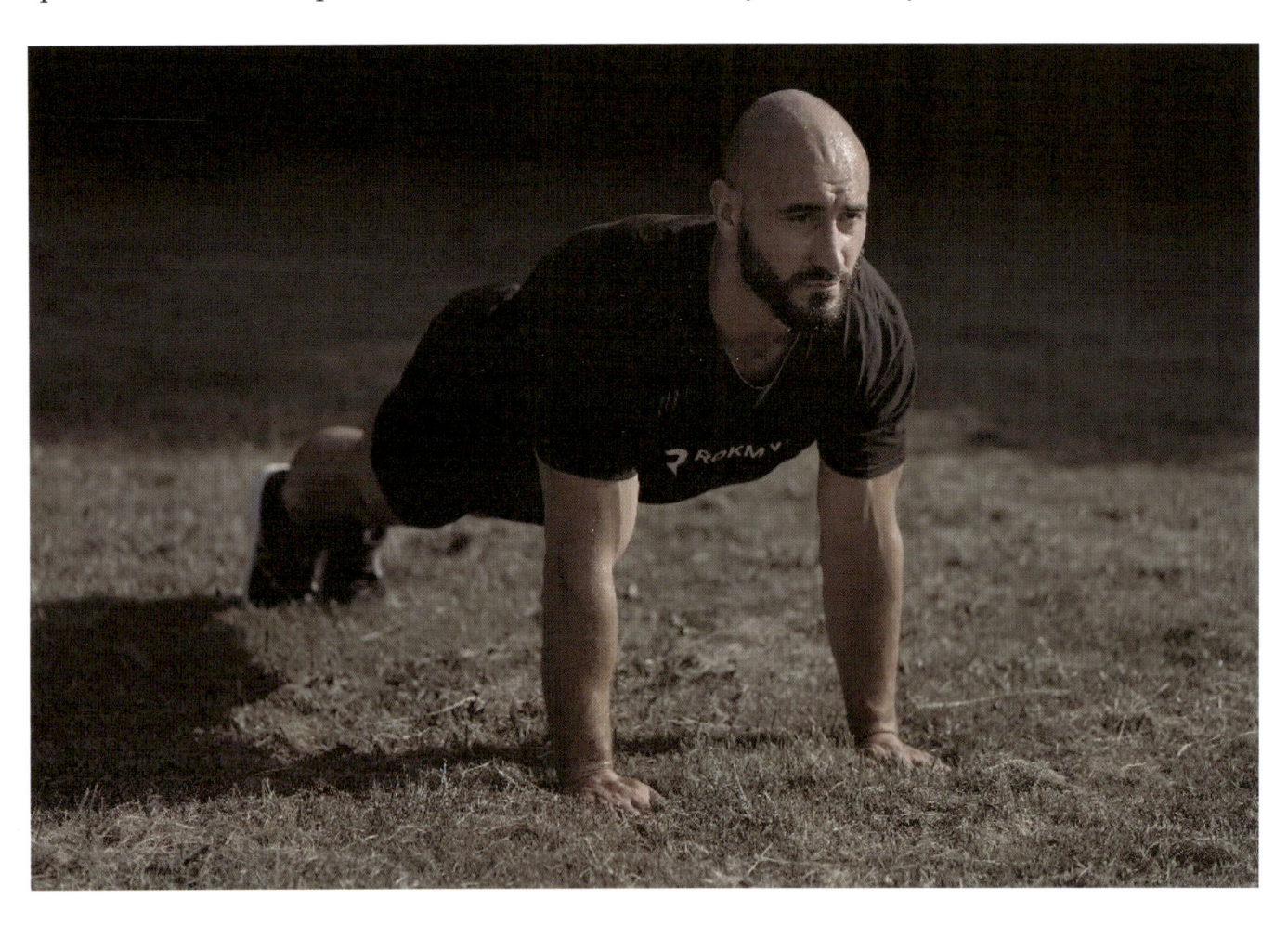

Hill Sprints

Hill sprints are an excellent way to quickly increase fitness, speed and stamina. They increase leg strength, power and conditioning. I would recommend using a hill with a 4-15% gradient. For individuals new to hill sprints, it would be advisable to start on the lower end and gradually build up.

For this programme, they are performed at a maximum effort with a distance that would take you approximately 30 seconds to travel. It is best to set out a target distance such as with a lamppost or other marker rather than going off time during the sprint as you should be focussing on running and not checking your gadgets.

Once you have completed your sprint, it is time to walk down the hill slowly and ensure that you are fully recovered before the next sprint I would suggest around 2 minutes rest between sprints. Repeat for the specified number of repetitions.

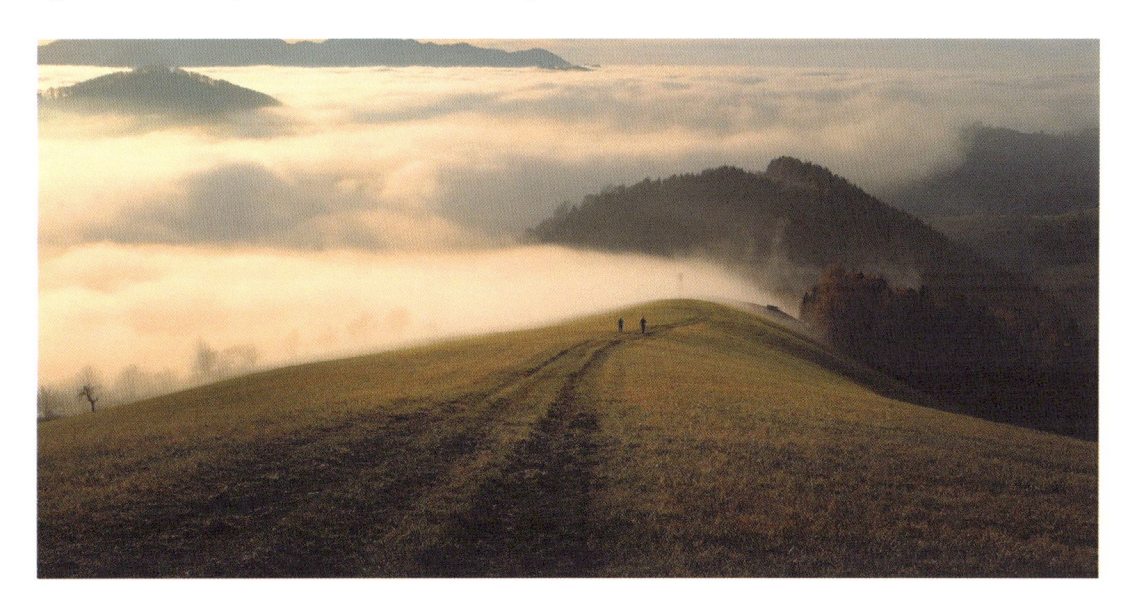

Steady Pace Runs

The aim of these runs is to build your endurance foundation and establish a baseline fitness, these are often referred to as "building the aerobic engine". The adaptations from this type of running occur over a longer period of time and so we are gradually increasing the distance, but the effort level should remain the same (you may find you start running quicker as the weeks go by but as long as the perceived effort level stays constant).

These runs are not designed to be hard. Use a pace that you would be able to maintain a conversation throughout and try and keep it constant throughout the whole run.

Moderate Pace Runs

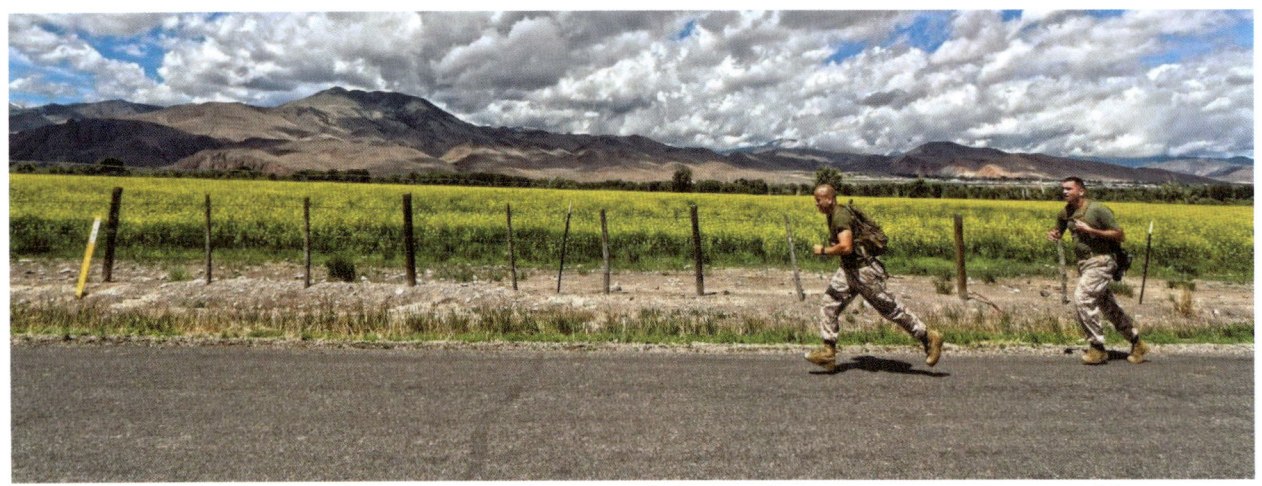

A step up from the steady pace run. The aim of the moderate pace run is to enable you to run faster for longer periods of time. It is a sustained effort for the specified distance that should be approaching uncomfortable, but still doable. You should still be able to talk.

Mobility and Dynamic Stretches

Here are some suggested mobility exercises that can be used as part of a daily mobility routine and your warm up. Performing these drills is a case of putting the joint through its range motion in a controlled manner and could help keep your joints healthy.

Mobility routine – repeat 10-30 times slow and controlled. Do not force the stretches.

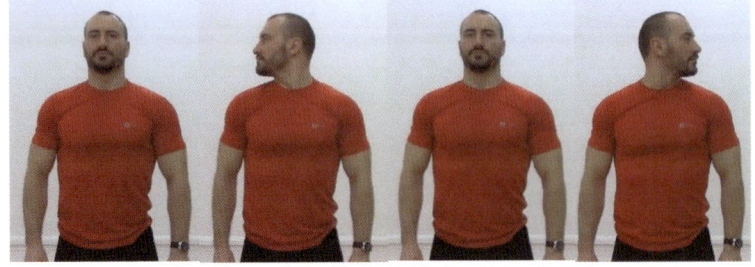

Stand tall and still, head facing the front.
Slowly turn your head from left to right whilst trying to keep the rest of your body still.

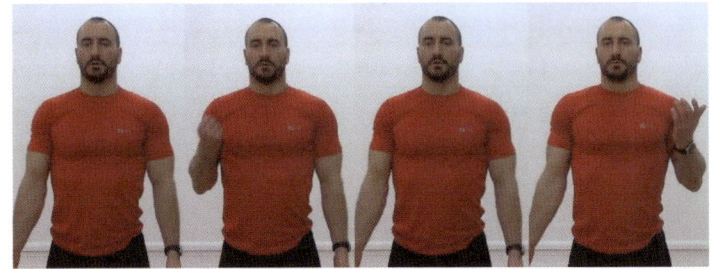

Slowly bend and straighten your arms
Stand tall and still
Keep the upper arm fixed in place

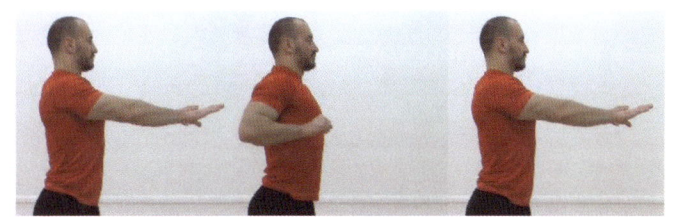

Stand tall and with good posture
Slowly bring your elbows back and then extend your arms forwards

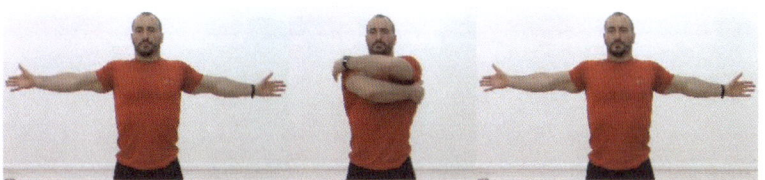

Wrap your arms around your body and then slowly stretch out to the sides

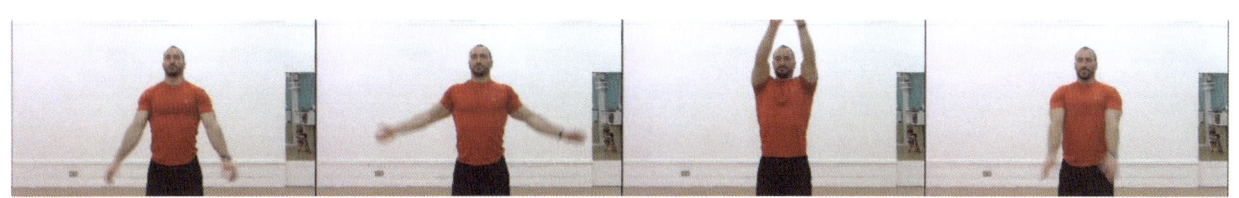

Large circles with your shoulders

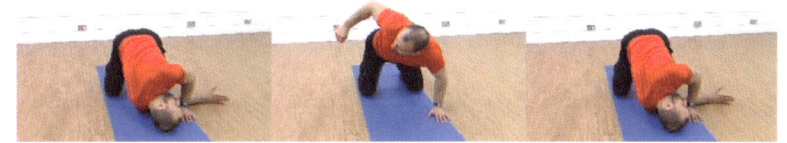

Keep your hips parallel to the floor and reach over to one side, then slowly rotate the trunk pointing one shoulder upwards

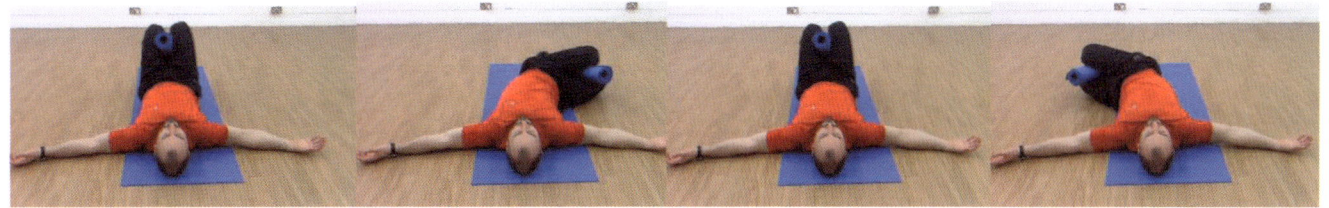

Lie on your back with a natural arch in the spine.
Bring your heels back and take a foam roller or rolled up mat between your legs.
Keep your shoulders on the floor and then slowly turn your pelvis and knee over to the side.
Then return to the centre and then over to the other side, then back to the centre.

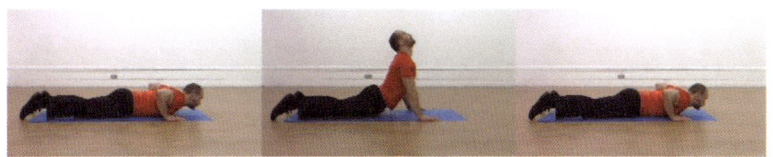

Lie on the floor with your hands below the shoulders and elbows tucked into the sides. Tense your glutes and slowly extend your arms and look upwards. Gently lower down.

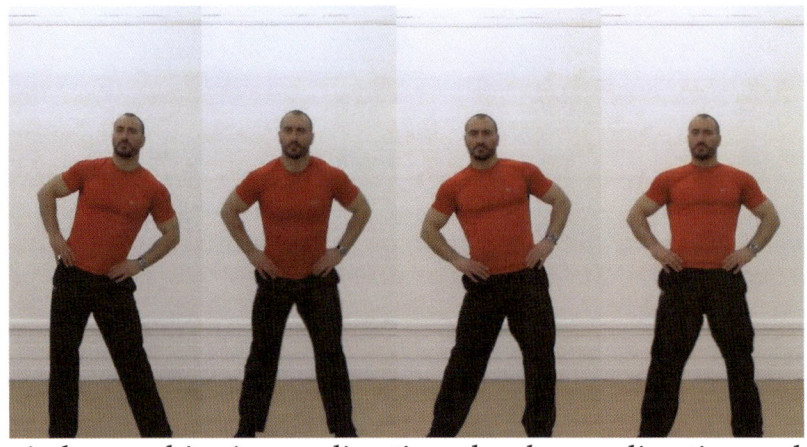

Slowly circle your hips in one direction, the change direction and repeat.

Warm Up Exercises

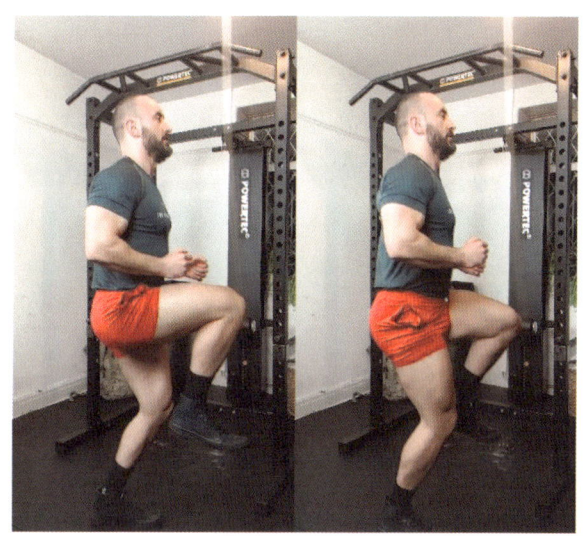

High knees – While running on the spot, lift your knees up and down alternating each side. Try and get your thighs parallel to the floor.

Perform for 30 seconds.

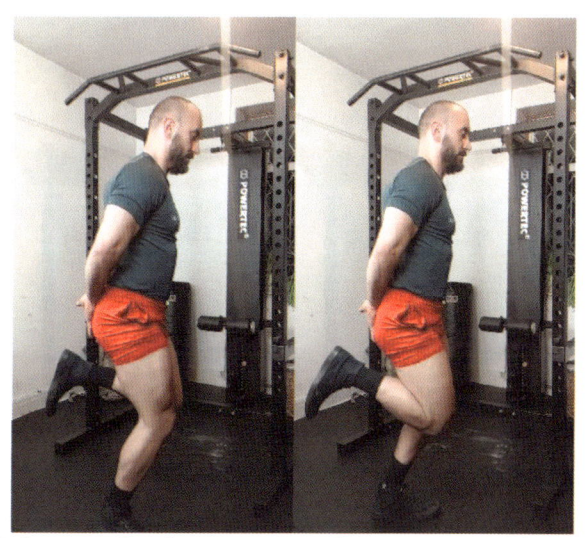

Heel Flicks - Flick your heels up towards your rear, alternating each side.

Perform for 30 seconds

Dynamic Hamstring Stretches

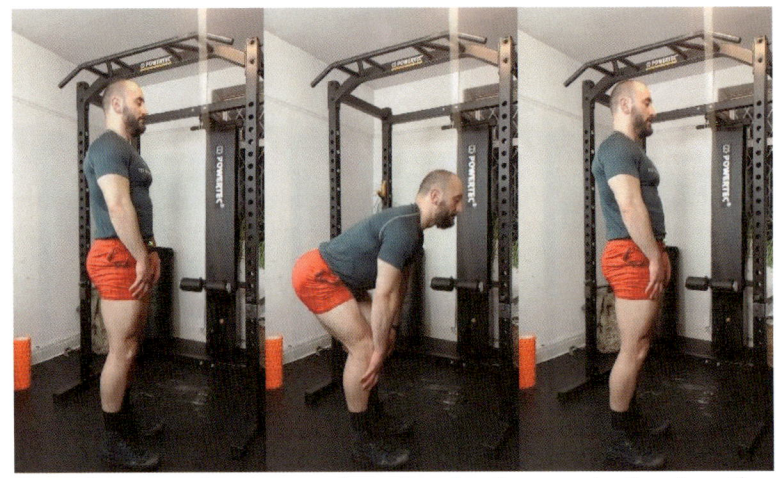

Stand tall with neutral spine and maintain the neutral spine throughout
Push your hips back bending your knees slightly until you feel a stretch on your hamstrings then push your hips forward to the starting position and tense your glutes.

Perform 15 repetitions

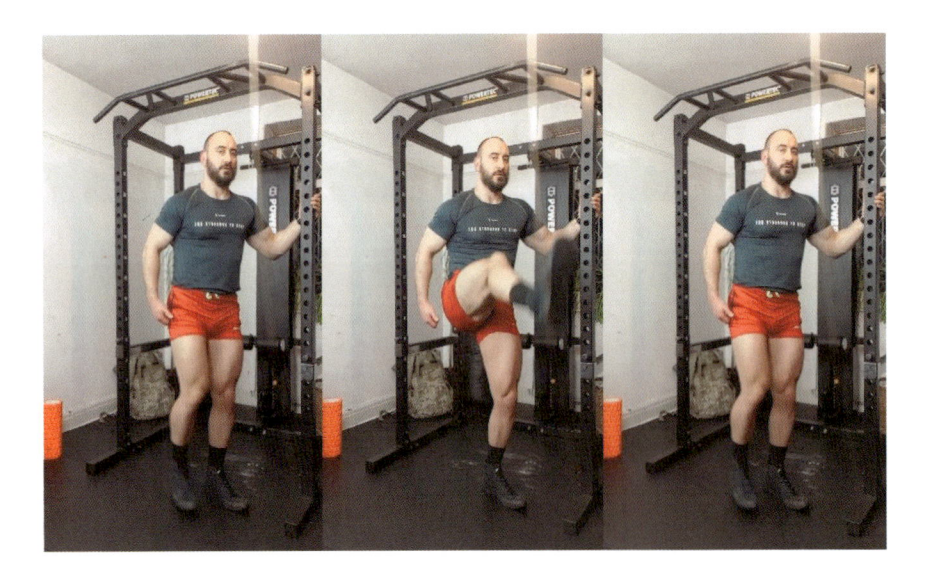

Kick your leg under control out to the front and try and keep straight. Go until you feel a stretch on your hamstring and them return the leg back to the starting position. Do not force the stretch.

Perform 15 repetitions each side

Exercises

Press Ups

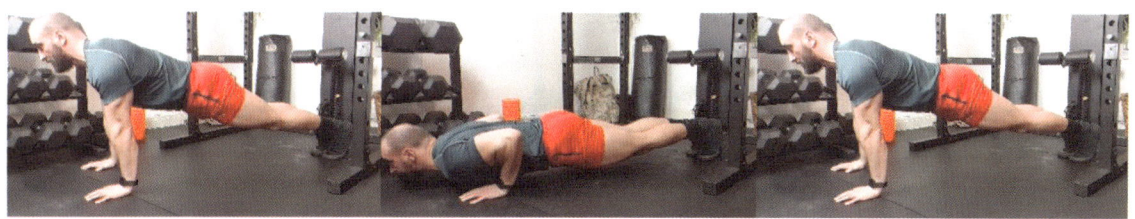

With your hands shoulder width apart, hands below the shoulders elbows towards the sides
1. Lower your chest to the floor, pivoting at the heel
2. Keep your body tight throughout
3. Full extend your arms

Press Ups with Knees Down

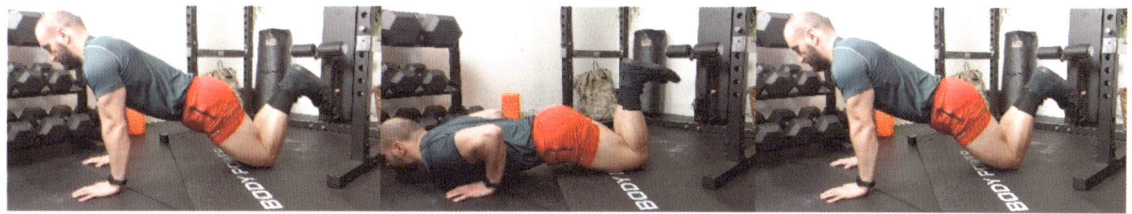

Same as above except knees are bent and on soft or cushioned floor such as a mat
1. Ensure the hips are forward of the knee

Body Row *Ensure the equipment you are using is sturdy so that you will not fall.*

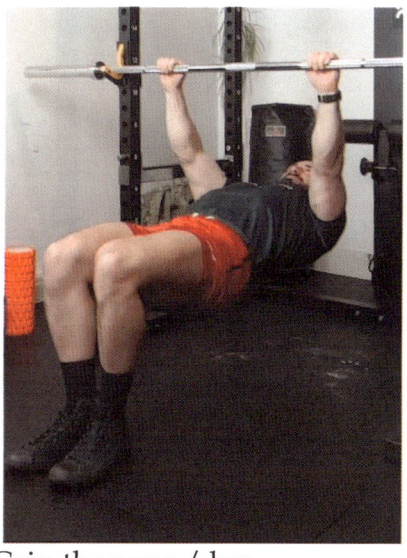

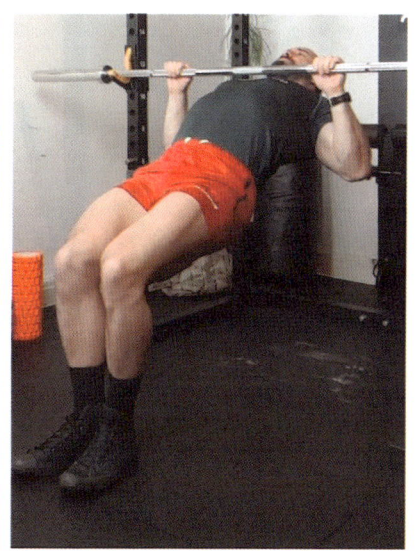

1. Grip the rope / bar
2. Keeping your legs either straight
3. Pull yourself up keeping your core tight and engaged
4. Pivot at the feet
5. Slowly lower yourself down
6. Repeat for desired number of repetitions

Burpee

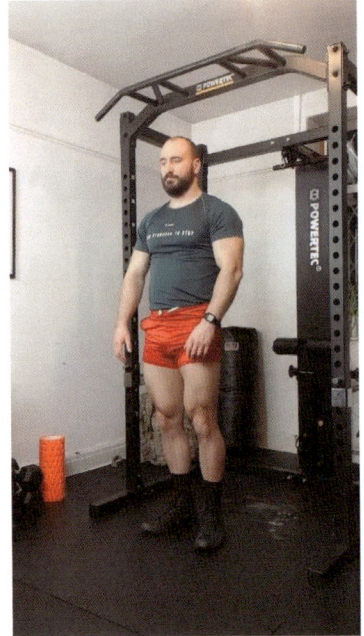

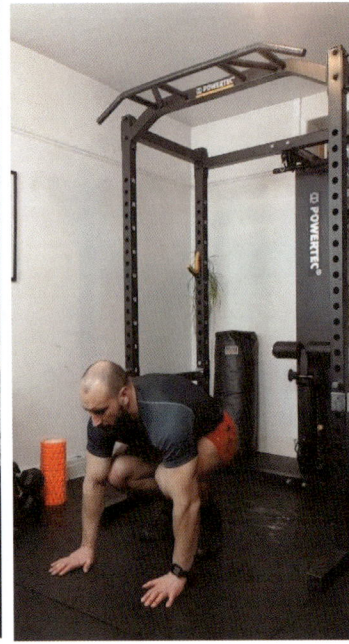

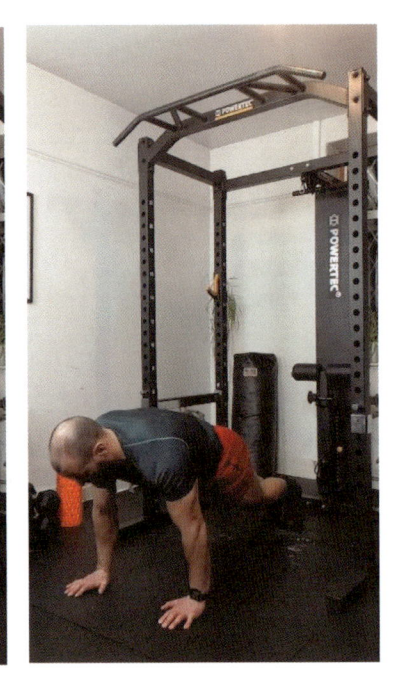

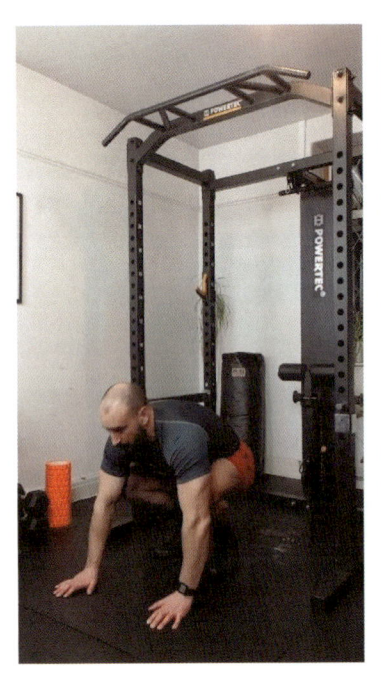

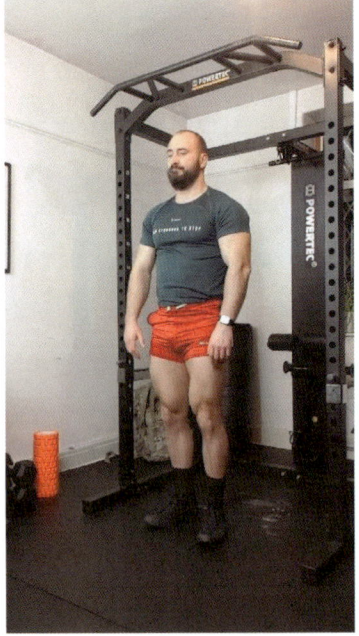

1. From a standing position bend at the knees bringing your hips towards the floor
2. Place your hands on the floor
3. Drive your legs back, full extending them
4. Keep your core engaged and tight throughout
5. Bring your knees back so you are in the squat position
6. Drive through the floor powerfully and extend your legs to return to the standing position
7. Repeat for desired number of repetitions

Squat

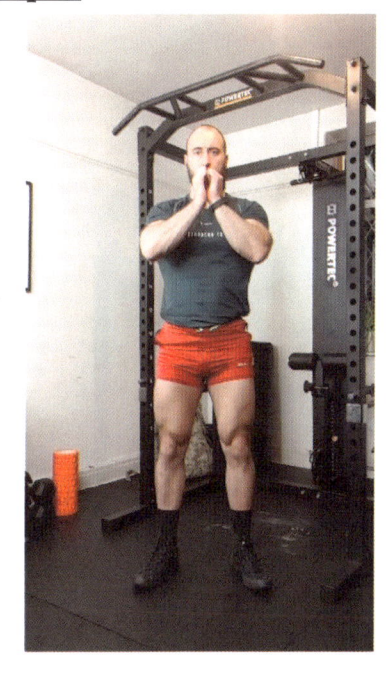

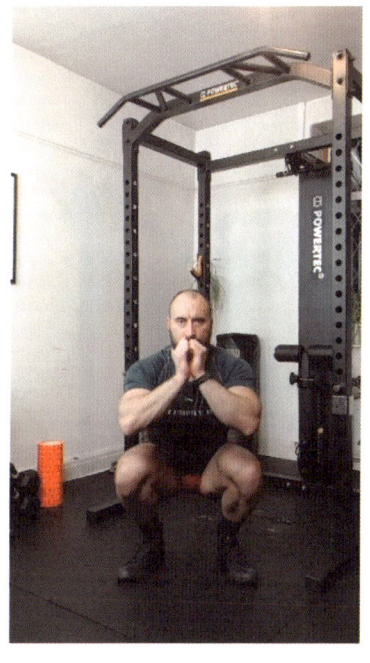

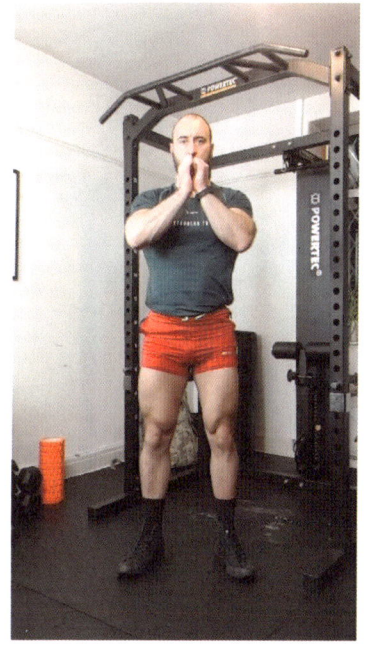

Stand tall with feet slightly wider than hip-width distance apart feet slightly turned out.

1. Look straight ahead and tighten your ab muscles
2. Bend your knees and sink your hips back while lowering your hips towards the floor. Try to keep a straight spine and tight core throughout the whole movement.
3. Straighten your legs and drive back up to standing position

Squats with dumbbell

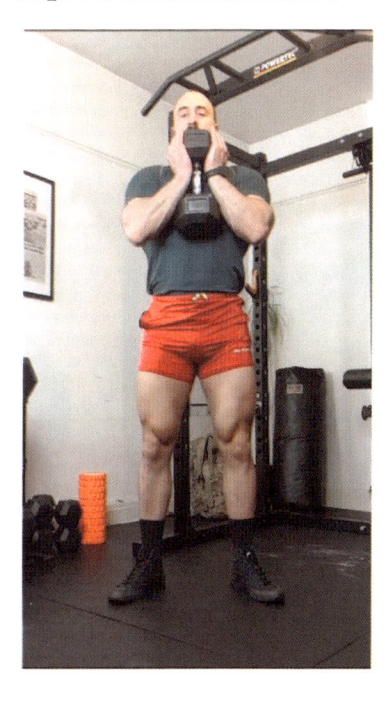

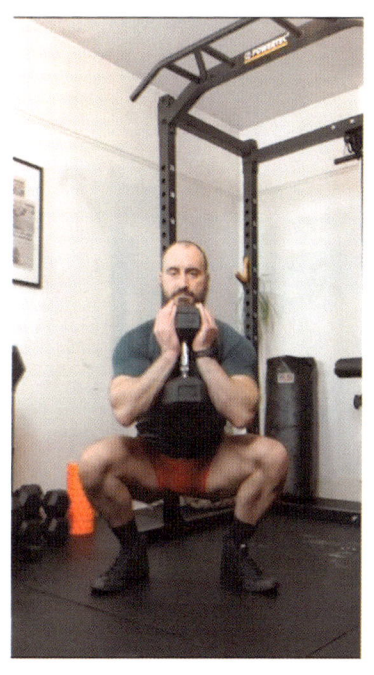

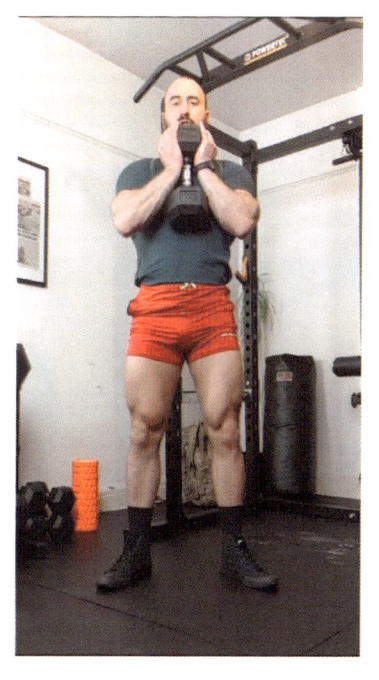

Squats with barbell

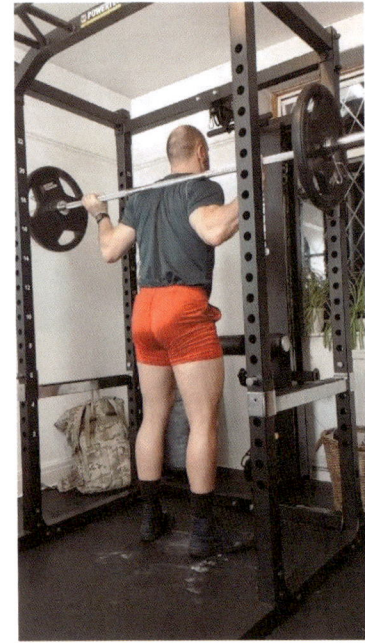

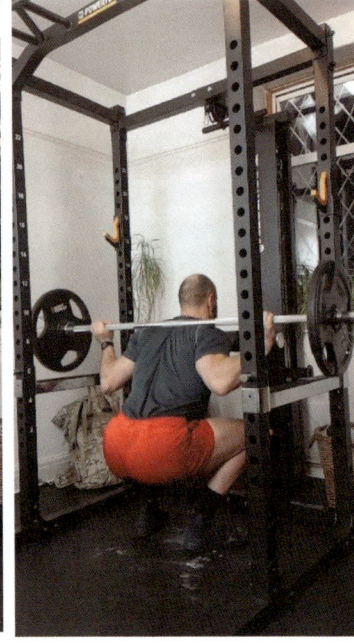

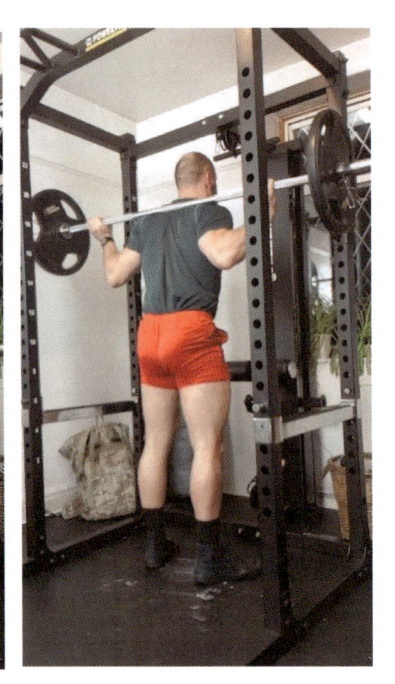

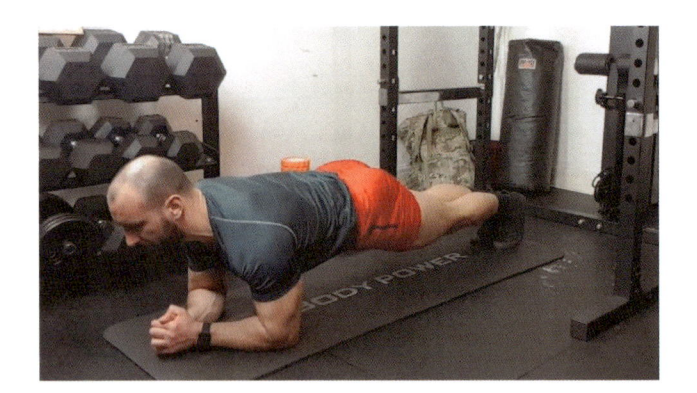

Plank
1. Elbows below the shoulder
2. Maintain a straight spine
3. Keep your core tight and engaged
4. Focus on your breathing

Lying Side Leg Lift

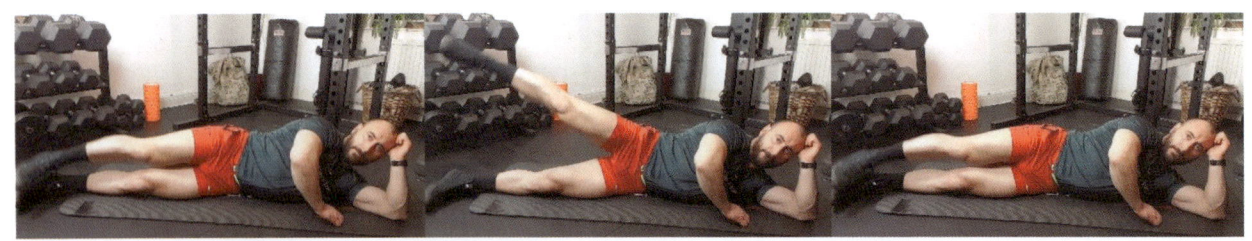

Lie on the side legs straight with your head supported by your hand
1. Slowly raise your top leg upwards, keep the side of your foot parallel to the floor
2. Slowly lower back down
3. Repeat for desired number of repetitions

Glute Bridge

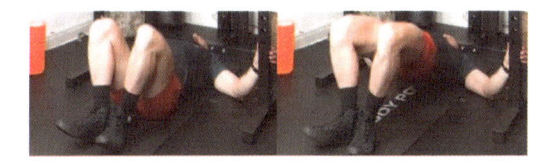

Keep neutral spine, shoulder and head flat on the floor. Bring heels back towards your butt and then drive the heels into the floor pushing your hips up and squeezing your glutes at the top of the movement, slowly lower down.

Single Leg Romanian Dead Lift

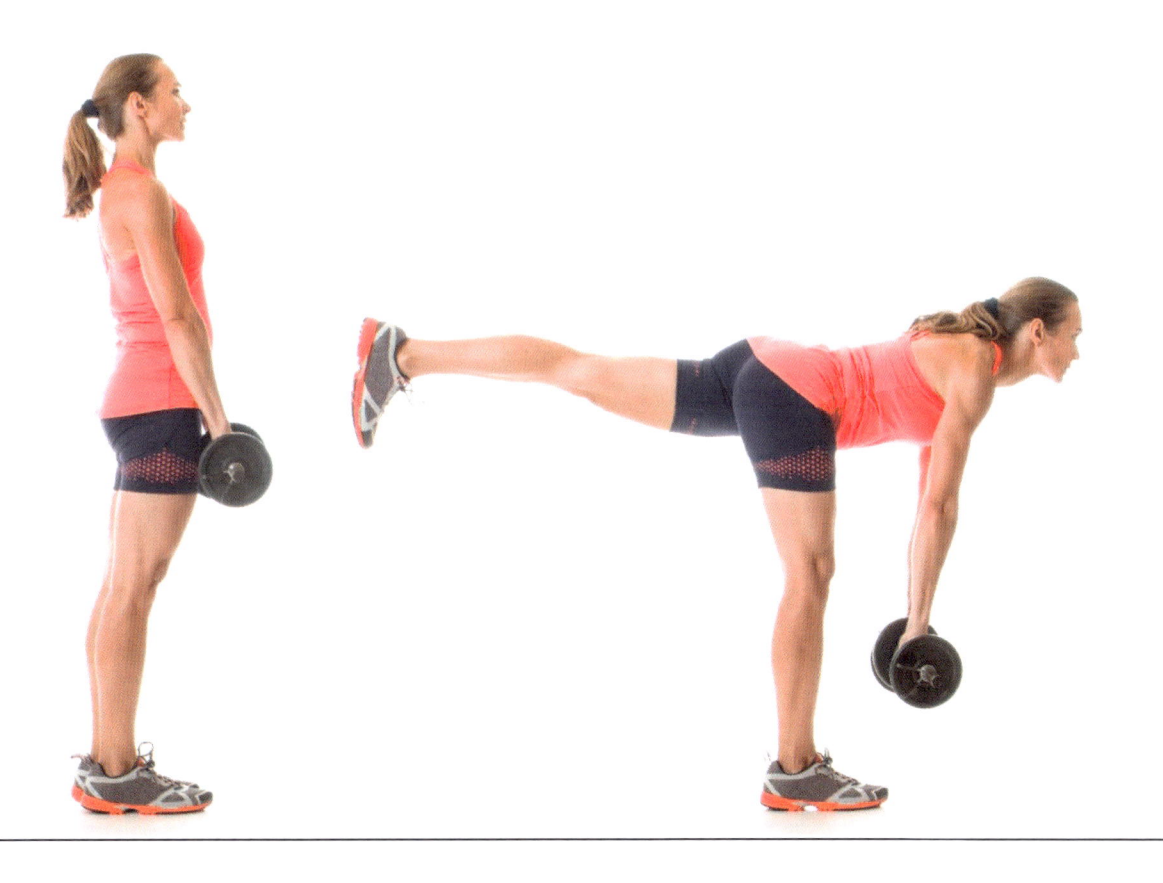

1. Stand tall and with a neutral spine
2. Lift one foot off the floor
3. Hinge at the hip, bending the knee slightly
4. Engage your glute and hamstring to return to the upright position
5. Repeat for desired number of reps

Can be performed with bodyweight only or with a dumbbell in the hands

Stretches

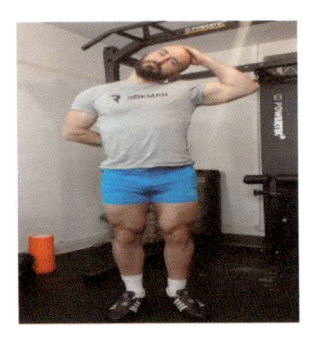

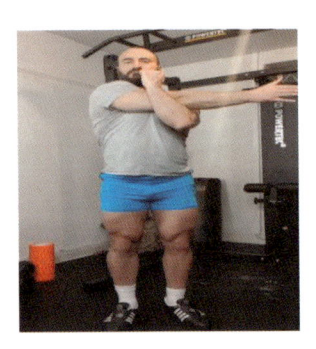

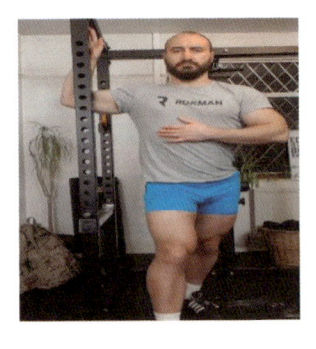

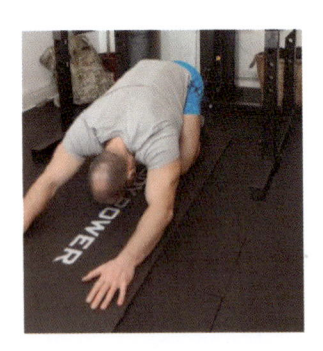

Trapezius Stretch
1. Stand upright looking straight ahead
2. Tilt your head to one side
3. Gently apply pressure with your hand until you feel the stretch on the side / rear of your neck
4. Hold for 30 seconds and repeat on the other side

Shoulder Stretch
1. Stand upright looking straight ahead
2. Bring your arm across your chest
3. Staying clear of the elbow joint, apply pressure with your other arm until you feel the stretch on your shoulder
4. Hold for 30 seconds and repeat on the other side

Chest Stretch
1. From a standing position place your forearm at an approximate right angle on a wall or squat rack frame
2. Gentle lean your bodyweight forwards until you feel a stretch on the chest
3. Hold for 30 seconds and repeat on the other side

Back Stretches
1. On all fours arms straight shoulders directly above the hands and hips above the knees
2. Gently sink your hip down towards your heels and reach your arms out to the front
3. Hold for 30 seconds and then ease out of the stretch to the starting position

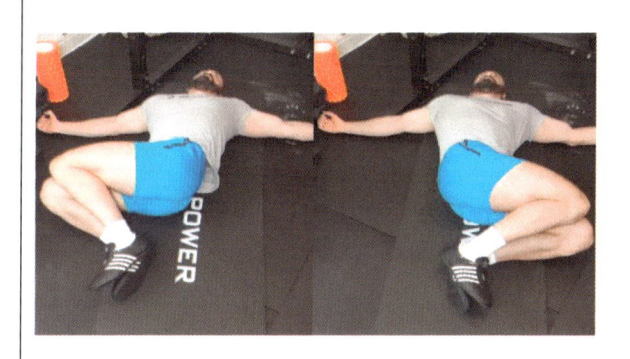

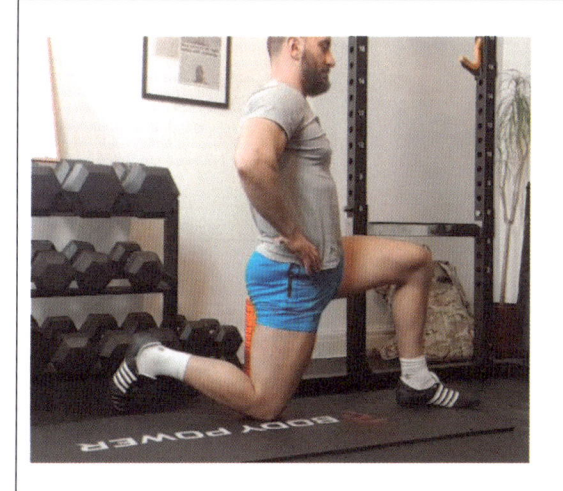

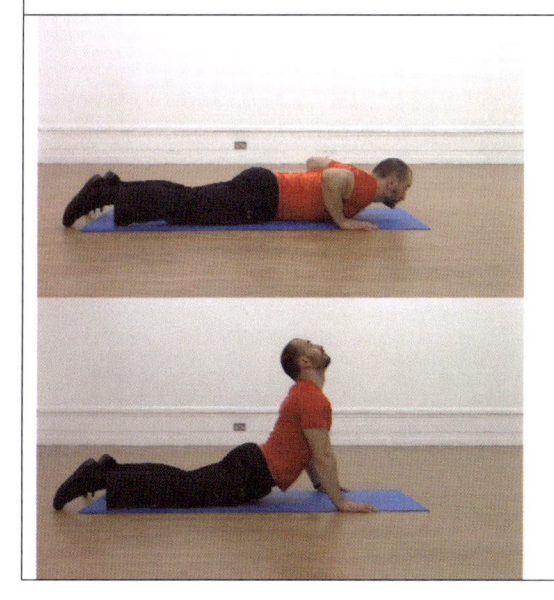

1. Start off lying on your back with head and shoulder on the floor
2. Bend the knees and slowly turn your pelvis to one side, keeping feet and knees together
3. Go until you feel the stretch and hold for 30 seconds and then repeat on the other side

Hip Flexor Stretch
1. Place your right knee on the floor and your left foot out to the front, slightly forward of the left knee
2. Tense your right glute as hard as you can throughout stretch
3. Slowly bring your hips forwards until your feel a stretch on the top of your right thigh
4. Hold for 30 seconds, ease backwards out of the stretch and repeat on the other side

Abdominal and Hip Flexor Stretch
1. Lie on your front, hands directly below the shoulders
2. Tense your glutes as hard as you can throughout the entire stretch
3. Slowly extend your arms as far as you comfortably can
4. Hold for 15-30 seconds
5. Slowly lower back down

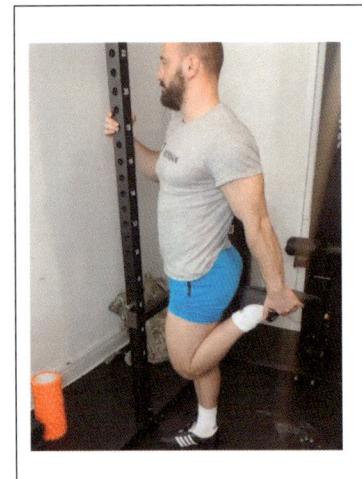

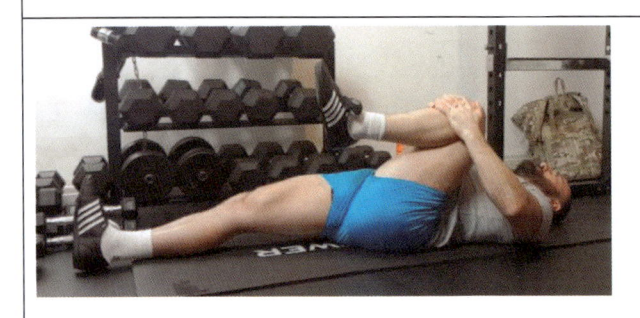

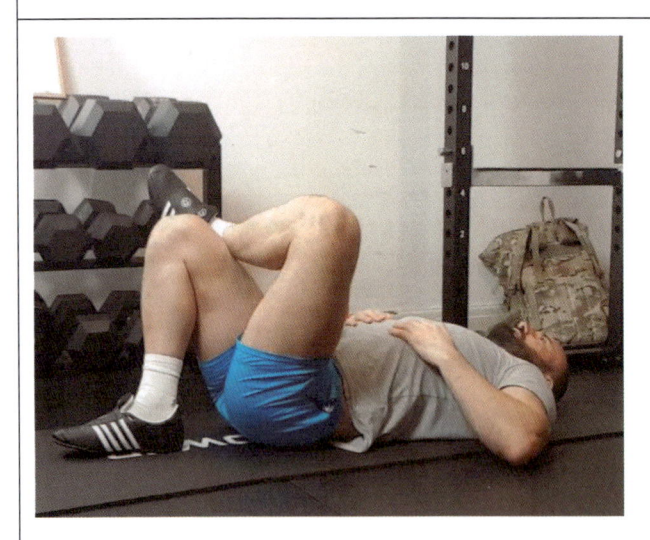

	Quadricep Stetch 1. From either a standing or lying position 2. Bend at the knee and take charge of your foot with you hand pulling your heel towards your glute 3. Keep knees in line and push the hips forward until you feel a stretch on the front of the thigh 4. Hold for 30 seconds and repeat on the other side
	Hamstring – Glute Stretch Routine 1. Lie on your back with both legs straight 2. Bring your left knee up towards your torso 3. Apply press on your shin to increase stretch 4. Hold for 30 seconds
	1. Release the above stretch 2. Bend your right knee and place foot flat on the floor 3. Bring your left foot inwards so the side of the left shin is rested on the right thigh just below the knee 4. Hold for 30 seconds to stretch the glute. 5. To increase the stretch, follow the below protocol, or; 6. Release the stretch and repeat this and the previous stretch on the opposite side

	1. From the above position
2. Place both hands on your right hamstring just below the knee and straighten your right leg pointing upwards towards the ceiling
3. Gently lean backwards until you feel an increased stretch on the left glute
4. Hold for 30 seconds and repeat the 3 stretches on the other side
	Hamstring Stretch
1. From a standing position
2. Step your right foot forwards keeping your right leg straight
3. Maintain a neutral spine, place your hands on the left thigh above the knee
4. Slowly sit back bending your leg knee and lowering your hips until your feel a stretch on the straight right leg
5. Hold for 30 seconds and repeat on the other side
	Calf Stretch
1. Face a wall or solid framed object such a squat rack
2. Place both hands on the wall (or frame as pictured)
3. With a staggered stance and both toes pointing forwards and heels on the floor
4. Slowly start to shift your hips forwards whilst firmly keeping your rear heel on the floor until your feel a stretch on your rear calf
5. Hold for 30 seconds, gently ease out of the stretch and repeat on the other side

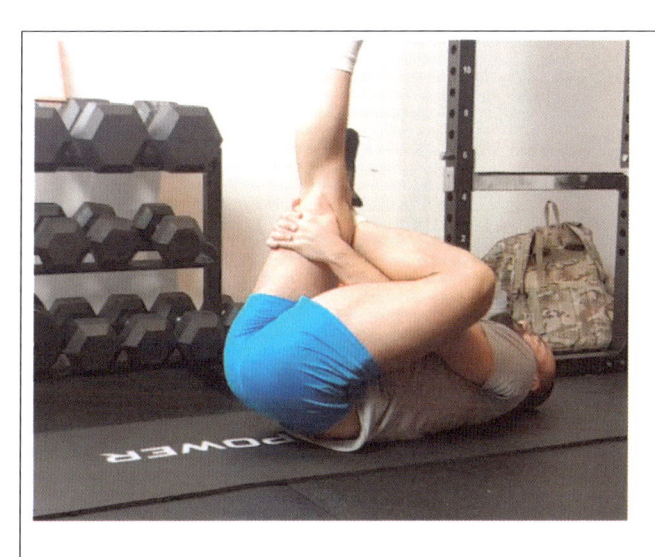

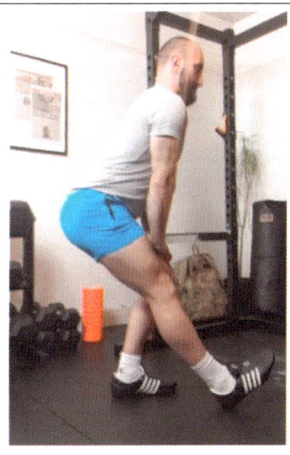

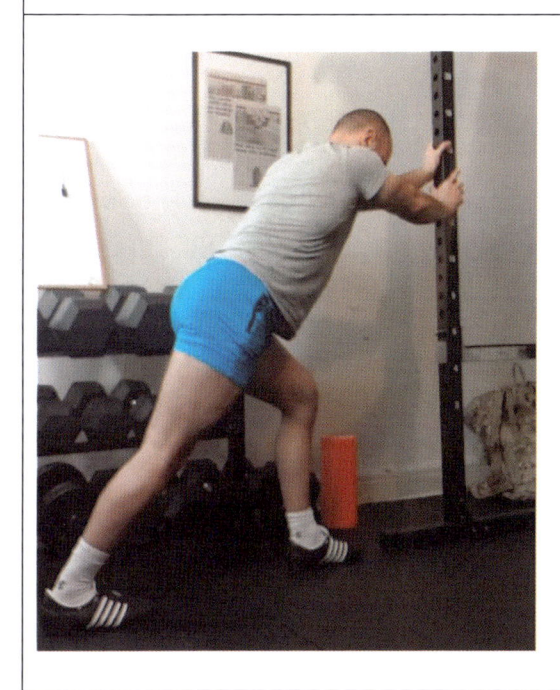

Testing

1.5 mile run
Aerobic Fitness Test. This is a 1.5 mile (2.4km) run test to measure the efficiency of your circulatory and respiratory system in supplying oxygen to your muscles during physical activity.

Spend 15 minutes warming up and then run 1.5 miles as quick as you can. This test is ideally performed on a running track; however, a treadmill can be used (1% gradient must be applied).

Rating	Time
Poor	>16:01
Fair	16:00-12:01
Good	12:00-10:31
Excellent	10:30-09:30
Superior	<09:29

Use the score sheet to make a log of your scores (the extra boxes are to allow you to use this programme multiple times if you wish to)

Date				
Your Time				
Target for next test (6 weeks' time)				

If you achieved the Poor or Fair rating you will now be assigned the rank of **Cadet** begin the Foundation Phase of the Commando Runner programme.

Good, Excellent and Superior will be accepted as **Recruits** and should jump straight into this level for the training programme.

However, if you feel you would benefit from the Foundation Phase of training then by all means you can do this.

You will notice in the foundation phase that the shortest run is 2 miles. If you are unable to run 3 miles without stopping then it is advisable to follow a developmental running plan to prepare you for the foundation phase.

This would consist of taking 4-8 weeks to gradually increase your running.

Perform 3 runs per week, spread out over the week for example Mon, Wed, Fri.

For the first few weeks do the following:

1. Establish a 2 mile route that is relatively flat
2. Walk / Run the route 3 times per week
3. Gradually aim to reduce the amount of walking you are doing, with the goal being to complete the 2 miles without having to stop
4. Use this period to practise your pace, keep it slow and steady

Once you can run 2 miles without needing to stop / walk, do this:

1. Establish a 3 mile route that is relatively flat
2. Maintain the same principles as above except now with the 3 mile course
3. The aim this time is to complete the 3 miles without having to stop

After you can run 3 miles without having to stop then do this:

1. Begin to practise your technique on the exercises as show in this programme
    a. Focus on quality – do them properly 2 sets of 10 repetitions would be fine to begin with
    b. Perform then on your days off running
2. Keep running your 3 miles, 3 times per week but change the route, include some small hills and inclines to make them a little bit more challenging

After you have completed this and are comfortable running 3 miles on flat and with some inclines thrown in then you will be in a better position to begin the Cadet Training Programme.

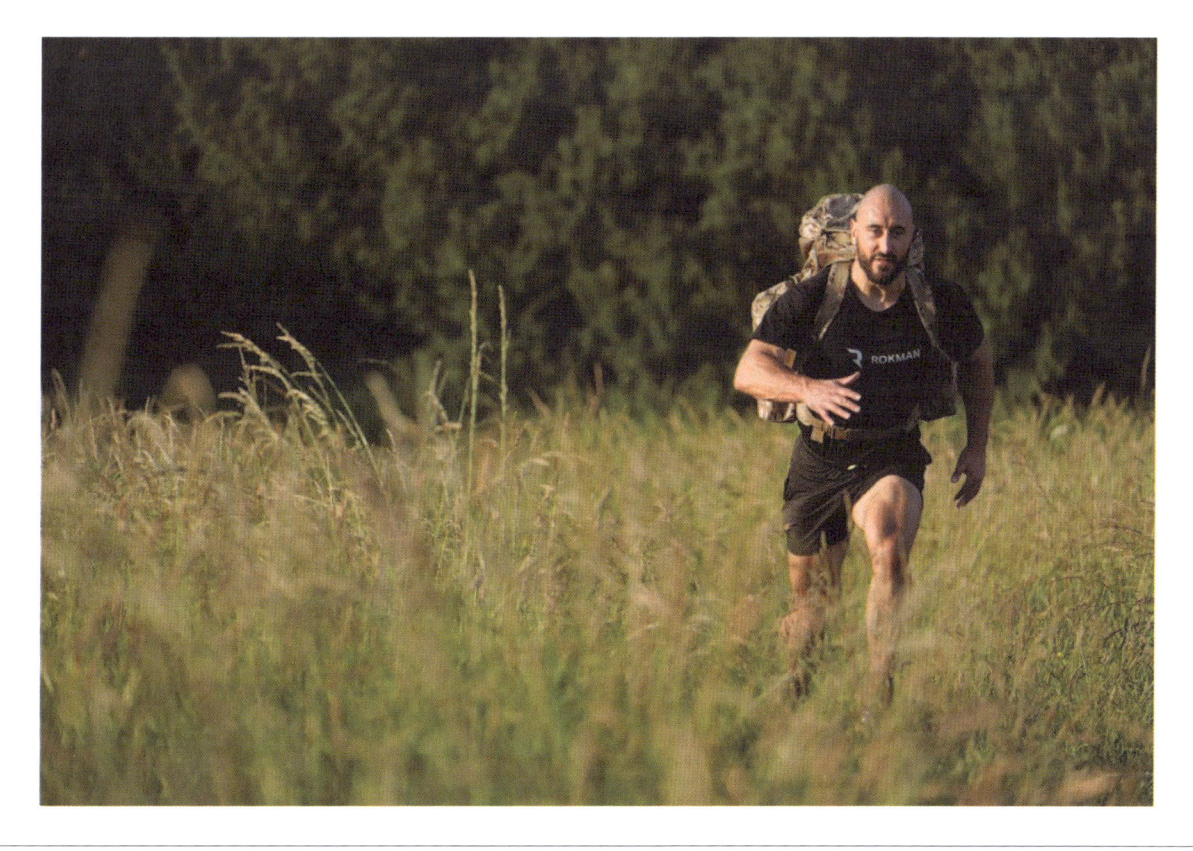

Cadet Training Programme Schedule

Foundation Phase

Day / Week	1	2	3	4	5	6	7
1	2 Mile Run	Walk	2 Mile Run + Strength	Walk	2 Mile Run	Strength	Rest
2	2.5 Mile Run	Walk	2.5 Mile Run + Strength	Walk	2.5 Mile Run	Strength	
3	3 Mile Run	Walk	3 Mile Run + Strength	Walk	3 Mile Run	Strength	Rest
4	3.5 Mile Run	Walk	3.5 Mile Run + Strength	Walk	3.5 Mile Run	Strength	Rest
5	4 Mile Run	Walk	4 Mile Run + Strength	Walk	4 Mile Run	Strength	Rest
6	4.5 Mile Run	Walk	4.5 Mile Run + Strength	Walk	4.5 Mile Run	Strength	Rest

Day by Day Training Programme
Example

Warm Up	
Briefing: Complete a 2 Mile run at a steady pace	**Stretches:** ✓ Work through the stretching guide
Time: 16.31	**Target for next session:** 16.15
Notes: Flat route, felt strong	

Sleep		
What time you went to bed: 2300	What time you woke up: 0700	Total hours sleep: 8

Day 1: 2 Mile Run

Warm Up
1 Minute of walking
3 Minutes of jogging at a slow pace
Mobility drills (high knees, heel flicks, hip circles)
10 side lying leg raises (each side)
10 glute bridges
1 Minute of jogging at a slow pace

Briefing: Complete a 2 Mile run at a steady pace	Stretches:
Time:	Target for next session:

Notes: *use this area to write any notes related to performance, session, how you are feeling etc*

Sleep		
What time you went to bed:	What time you woke up:	Total hours sleep:

Day 2: Walk

Briefing: Complete a 40-60 minute walk 10 x side lying leg raises (each side) 10 glute bridges	Stretches:

Notes:

Sleep		
What time you went to bed:	What time you woke up:	Total hours sleep:

Day 3: 2 Mile Run + Strength

Warm Up	
1 Minute of walking 3 Minutes of jogging at a slow pace Mobility drills (high knees, heel flicks, hip circles) 10 side lying leg raises (each side) 10 glute bridges 1 Minute of jogging at a slow pace	
Briefing: Complete a 2 Mile run at a steady pace followed by a strength circuit: Squats x 20 Press ups x 10 Single Leg Romanian Dead lifts x 10 (each side) Plank 30 seconds Body Row x 12	**Stretches:**
Time:	**Target for next session:**
Notes:	

Sleep		
What time you went to bed:	What time you woke up:	Total hours sleep:

Day 4: Walk

Briefing: Complete a 40-60 minute walk 10 x side lying leg raises (each side) 10 glute bridges	**Stretches:**
Notes:	

Sleep		
What time you went to bed:	What time you woke up:	Total hours sleep:

Day 5: 2 Mile Run

Warm Up
1 Minute of walking
3 Minutes of jogging at a slow pace
Mobility drills (high knees, heel flicks, hip circles)
10 side lying leg raises (each side)
10 glute bridges
1 Minute of jogging at a slow pace

Briefing: Complete a 2 Mile run at a steady pace	Stretches:
Time:	Target for next session:
Notes:	

Sleep		
What time you went to bed:	What time you woke up:	Total hours sleep:

Day 6: Strength

Warm Up
1 Minute of walking
3 Minutes of jogging at a slow pace
Mobility drills (high knees, heel flicks, hip circles)
10 side lying leg raises (each side)
10 glute bridges
1 Minute of jogging at a slow pace
Alternatively, you can use a cross trainer or a rower to warm up for 5 minutes, but still perform the mobility drills and activation exercises

Briefing: Complete 2 rounds of the circuit	Stretches:
Squats x 20	
Press ups x 10	
Single Leg Romanian Dead lifts x 10 (each side)	
Plank 30 seconds	
Body Row x 12	
Time:	Target for next session:
Notes:	

Sleep		
What time you went to bed:	What time you woke up:	Total hours sleep:

Day 7: Rest

Briefing: Rest and relax. Do not do anything intense on this day. Gentle walk, swimming, mobility drills are OK and recommended.

Notes: Reflect on the progress you have made this week. Think about what you are going to achieve over the next week.

Sleep		
What time you went to bed:	What time you woke up:	Total hours sleep:

Day 8: 2.5 Mile Run

Warm Up
1 Minute of walking
3 Minutes of jogging at a slow pace
Mobility drills (high knees, heel flicks, hip circles)
10 side lying leg raises (each side)
10 glute bridges
1 Minute of jogging at a slow pace

Briefing: Complete a 2.5 Mile run at a steady pace	**Stretches:**
Time:	**Target for next session:**

Notes: use this area to write any notes related to performance, session, how you are feeling etc

Sleep		
What time you went to bed:	What time you woke up:	Total hours sleep:

Day 9: Walk

Briefing: Complete a 40-60 minute walk 10 x side lying leg raises (each side) 10 glute bridges	Stretches:
Notes:	

Sleep		
What time you went to bed:	What time you woke up:	Total hours sleep:

Day 10: 2.5 Mile Run + Strength

Warm Up
1 Minute of walking
3 Minutes of jogging at a slow pace
Mobility drills (high knees, heel flicks, hip circles)
10 side lying leg raises (each side)
10 glute bridges
1 Minute of jogging at a slow pace

Briefing: Complete a 2 Mile run at a steady pace followed by a strength circuit: Squats x 22 Press ups x 12 Single Leg Romanian Dead lifts x 12 (each side) Plank 45 seconds Body Row x 14	Stretches:
Time:	**Target for next session:**
Notes:	

Sleep		
What time you went to bed:	What time you woke up:	Total hours sleep:

Day 11: Walk

Briefing: Complete a 50-70 minute walk 10 x side lying leg raises (each side) 10 glute bridges	Stretches:
Notes: *use this area to write any notes related to performance, session, how you are feeling etc*	

Sleep		
What time you went to bed:	What time you woke up:	Total hours sleep:

Day 12: 2.5 Mile Run

Warm Up
1 Minute of walking
3 Minutes of jogging at a slow pace
Mobility drills (high knees, heel flicks, hip circles)
10 side lying leg raises (each side)
10 glute bridges
1 Minute of jogging at a slow pace

Briefing: Complete a 2.5 Mile run at a steady pace	Stretches:
Time:	Target for next session:
Notes: *use this area to write any notes related to performance, session, how you are feeling etc*	

Sleep		
What time you went to bed:	What time you woke up:	Total hours sleep:

Day 13: Strength

Warm Up
1 Minute of walking
3 Minutes of jogging at a slow pace
Mobility drills (high knees, heel flicks, hip circles)
10 side lying leg raises (each side)
10 glute bridges
1 Minute of jogging at a slow pace
Alternatively, you can use a cross trainer or a rower to warm up for 5 minutes, but still perform the mobility drills and activation exercises

Briefing: Complete 2 rounds of the circuit Squats x 22 Press ups x 12 Single Leg Romanian Dead lifts x 12 (each side) Plank 45 seconds Body Row x 12	Stretches:
Time:	Target for next session:

Notes:

Sleep

What time you went to bed:	What time you woke up:	Total hours sleep:

Day 14: Rest

Briefing: Rest and relax. Do not do anything intense on this day. Gentle walk, swimming, mobility drills are OK and recommended.

Notes: *Reflect on the progress you have made this week. Think about what you are going to achieve over the next week.*

Sleep

What time you went to bed:	What time you woke up:	Total hours sleep:

Day 15: 3 Mile Run

Warm Up
1 Minute of walking
3 Minutes of jogging at a slow pace
Mobility drills (high knees, heel flicks, hip circles)
10 side lying leg raises (each side)
10 glute bridges
1 Minute of jogging at a slow pace

Briefing: Complete a 3 Mile run at a steady pace	Stretches:
Time:	Target for next session:

Notes: use this area to write any notes related to performance, session, how you are feeling etc

Sleep		
What time you went to bed:	What time you woke up:	Total hours sleep:

Day 16: Walk

Briefing: Complete a 50-70 minute walk 10 x side lying leg raises (each side) 10 glute bridges	Stretches:

Notes: use this area to write any notes related to performance, session, how you are feeling etc

Sleep		
What time you went to bed:	What time you woke up:	Total hours sleep:

Day 17: 3 Mile Run + Strength

Warm Up
1 Minute of walking
3 Minutes of jogging at a slow pace
Mobility drills (high knees, heel flicks, hip circles)
10 side lying leg raises (each side)
10 glute bridges
1 Minute of jogging at a slow pace

Briefing: Complete a 3 Mile run at a steady pace followed by a strength circuit: Squats x 24 Press ups x 14 Single Leg Romanian Dead lifts x 14 (each side) Plank 60 seconds Body Row x 16	Stretches:
Time:	Target for next session:
Notes:	

Sleep		
What time you went to bed:	What time you woke up:	Total hours sleep:

Day 18: Walk

Fun fact
Most people have given up on a training programme by now. Have you got what it takes to succeed?

Briefing: Complete a 50-70 minute walk 10 x side lying leg raises (each side) 10 glute bridges	Stretches:
Notes:	

Sleep		
What time you went to bed:	What time you woke up:	Total hours sleep:

Day 19: 3 Mile Run

Warm Up
1 Minute of walking
3 Minutes of jogging at a slow pace
Mobility drills (high knees, heel flicks, hip circles)
10 side lying leg raises (each side)
10 glute bridges
1 Minute of jogging at a slow pace

Briefing: Complete a 3 Mile run at a steady pace	Stretches:
Time:	Target for next session:
Notes:	

Sleep		
What time you went to bed:	What time you woke up:	Total hours sleep:

Day 20: Strength

Warm Up
1 Minute of walking
3 Minutes of jogging at a slow pace
Mobility drills (high knees, heel flicks, hip circles)
12 side lying leg raises (each side)
12 glute bridges
1 Minute of jogging at a slow pace
Alternatively, you can use a cross trainer or a rower to warm up for 5 minutes, but still perform the mobility drills and activation exercises

Briefing: Complete 2 rounds of the circuit Squats x 24 Press ups x 14 Single Leg Romanian Dead lifts x 14 (each side) Plank 60 seconds Body Row x 14	Stretches:
Time:	Target for next session:
Notes: use this area to write any notes related to performance, session, how you are feeling etc	

Sleep		
What time you went to bed:	What time you woke up:	Total hours sleep:

Day 21: Rest

Briefing: Rest and relax. Do not do anything intense on this day. Gentle walk, swimming, mobility drills are OK and recommended.

Notes: *Reflect on the progress you have made this week. Think about what you are going to achieve over the next week.*

Sleep

What time you went to bed:	What time you woke up:	Total hours sleep:

Day 22: 3.5 Mile Run

Warm Up
1 Minute of walking
3 Minutes of jogging at a slow pace
Mobility drills (high knees, heel flicks, hip circles)
12 side lying leg raises (each side)
12 glute bridges
1 Minute of jogging at a slow pace

Briefing: Complete a 3.5 Mile run at a steady pace	Stretches:
Time:	Target for next session:

Notes: *use this area to write any notes related to performance, session, how you are feeling etc*

Sleep

What time you went to bed:	What time you woke up:	Total hours sleep:

Day 23: Walk

Briefing: Complete a 50-70 minute walk 12 side lying leg raises (each side) 12 glute bridges	Stretches:
Notes:	

Sleep		
What time you went to bed:	What time you woke up:	Total hours sleep:

Day 24: 3.5 Mile Run + Strength

Warm Up 1 Minute of walking 3 Minutes of jogging at a slow pace Mobility drills (high knees, heel flicks, hip circles) 12 side lying leg raises (each side) 12 glute bridges 1 Minute of jogging at a slow pace	
Briefing: Complete a 3.5 Mile run at a steady pace followed by a strength circuit: Squats x 25 Press ups x 15 Single Leg Romanian Dead lifts x 15 (each side) Plank 60 seconds Body Row x 17	Stretches:
Time:	**Target for next session:**
Notes: *use this area to write any notes related to performance, session, how you are feeling etc*	

Sleep		
What time you went to bed:	What time you woke up:	Total hours sleep:

Day 25: Walk

Briefing: Complete a 60-90 minute walk 15 side lying leg raises (each side) 15 glute bridges	Stretches:
Notes: *use this area to write any notes related to performance, session, how you are feeling etc*	
Sleep	
What time you went to bed:	What time you woke up:	Total hours sleep:

Day 26: 3.5 Mile Run

Warm Up
1 Minute of walking
3 Minutes of jogging at a slow pace
Mobility drills (high knees, heel flicks, hip circles)
15 side lying leg raises (each side)
15 glute bridges
1 Minute of jogging at a slow pace

Briefing: Complete a 3.5 Mile run at a steady pace	Stretches:
Time:	Target for next session:
Notes: *use this area to write any notes related to performance, session, how you are feeling etc*	
Sleep	
What time you went to bed:	What time you woke up:	Total hours sleep:

Day 27: Strength

Warm Up
1 Minute of walking
3 Minutes of jogging at a slow pace
Mobility drills (high knees, heel flicks, hip circles)
15 side lying leg raises (each side)
15 glute bridges
1 Minute of jogging at a slow pace
Alternatively, you can use a cross trainer or a rower to warm up for 5 minutes, but still perform the mobility drills and activation exercises

Briefing: Complete 2 rounds of the circuit	Stretches:
Squats x 25	
Press ups x 15	
Single Leg Romanian Dead lifts x 15 (each side)	
Plank 60 seconds	
Body Row x 17	
Time:	**Target for next session:**

Notes: *use this area to write any notes related to performance, session, how you are feeling etc*

Sleep		
What time you went to bed:	What time you woke up:	Total hours sleep:

Day 28: Rest

Briefing: Rest and relax. Do not do anything intense on this day. Gentle walk, swimming, mobility drills are OK and recommended.

Notes: *Reflect on the progress you have made this week. Think about what you are going to achieve over the next week.*

Sleep		
What time you went to bed:	What time you woke up:	Total hours sleep:

Day 29: 4 Mile Run

Warm Up
1 Minute of walking
3 Minutes of jogging at a slow pace
Mobility drills (high knees, heel flicks, hip circles)
16 side lying leg raises (each side)
16 glute bridges
1 Minute of jogging at a slow pace

Briefing: Complete a 4 Mile run at a steady pace	Stretches:
Time:	Target for next session:

Notes: use this area to write any notes related to performance, session, how you are feeling etc

Sleep		
What time you went to bed:	What time you woke up:	Total hours sleep:

Day 30: Walk

Briefing: Complete a 60-90 minute walk 16 side lying leg raises (each side) 16 glute bridges	Stretches:

Notes: use this area to write any notes related to performance, session, how you are feeling etc

Sleep		
What time you went to bed:	What time you woke up:	Total hours sleep:

Day 31: 4 Mile Run + Strength

Warm Up	
1 Minute of walking 3 Minutes of jogging at a slow pace Mobility drills (high knees, heel flicks, hip circles) 16 side lying leg raises (each side) 16 glute bridges 1 Minute of jogging at a slow pace	
Briefing: Complete a 4 Mile run at a steady pace followed by a strength circuit: Squats x 26 Press ups x 16 Single Leg Romanian Dead lifts x 16 (each side) Plank 60 seconds Body Row x 18	**Stretches:**
Time:	**Target for next session:**
Notes: use this area to write any notes related to performance, session, how you are feeling etc	
Sleep		
What time you went to bed:	What time you woke up:	Total hours sleep:

Day 32: Walk

Briefing: Complete a 60-90 minute walk 16 side lying leg raises (each side) 16 glute bridges	**Stretches:**
Notes: use this area to write any notes related to performance, session, how you are feeling etc	
Sleep		
What time you went to bed:	What time you woke up:	Total hours sleep:

Day 33: 4 Mile Run

Warm Up
1 Minute of walking
3 Minutes of jogging at a slow pace
Mobility drills (high knees, heel flicks, hip circles)
16 side lying leg raises (each side)
16 glute bridges
1 Minute of jogging at a slow pace

Briefing: Complete a 4 Mile run at a steady pace	Stretches:
Time:	Target for next session:

Notes: use this area to write any notes related to performance, session, how you are feeling etc

Sleep		
What time you went to bed:	What time you woke up:	Total hours sleep:

Keep Going

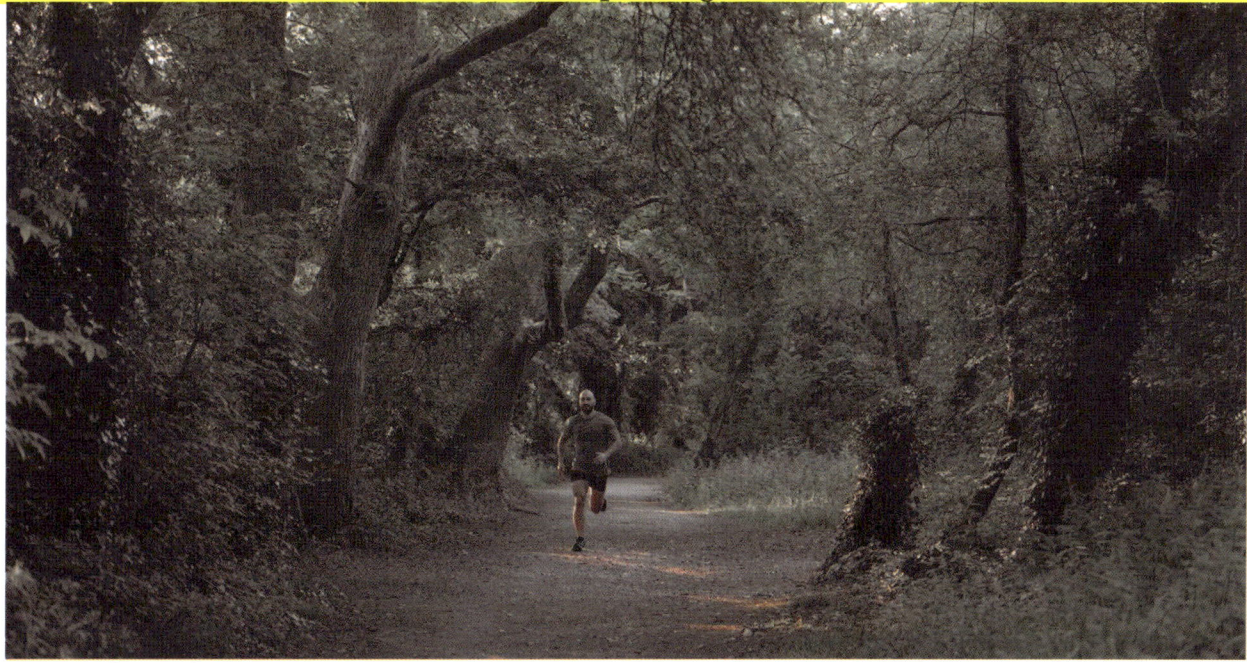

Image credit: Rokman

Day 34: Strength

Warm Up
1 Minute of walking
3 Minutes of jogging at a slow pace
Mobility drills (high knees, heel flicks, hip circles)
17 side lying leg raises (each side)
17 glute bridges
1 Minute of jogging at a slow pace
Alternatively, you can use a cross trainer or a rower to warm up for 5 minutes, but still perform the mobility drills and activation exercises

Briefing: Complete 2 rounds of the circuit	Stretches:
Squats x 26	
Press ups x 16	
Single Leg Romanian Dead lifts x 16 (each side)	
Plank 60 seconds	
Body Row x 18	
Time:	**Target for next session:**

Notes: *use this area to write any notes related to performance, session, how you are feeling etc*

Sleep		
What time you went to bed:	What time you woke up:	Total hours sleep:

Day 35: Rest

Briefing: Rest and relax. Do not do anything intense on this day. Gentle walk, swimming, mobility drills are OK and recommended.

Notes: *Reflect on the progress you have made this week. Think about what you are going to achieve over the next week.*

Sleep		
What time you went to bed:	What time you woke up:	Total hours sleep:

Day 36: 4.5 Mile Run

Warm Up
1 Minute of walking
3 Minutes of jogging at a slow pace
Mobility drills (high knees, heel flicks, hip circles)
17 side lying leg raises (each side)
17 glute bridges
1 Minute of jogging at a slow pace

Briefing: Complete a 4.5 Mile run at a steady pace	Stretches:
Time:	Target for next session:

Notes: use this area to write any notes related to performance, session, how you are feeling etc

Sleep		
What time you went to bed:	What time you woke up:	Total hours sleep:

Day 37: Walk

Briefing: Complete a 60-90 minute walk 16 side lying leg raises (each side) 16 glute bridges	Stretches:

Notes: use this area to write any notes related to performance, session, how you are feeling etc

Sleep		
What time you went to bed:	What time you woke up:	Total hours sleep:

Day 38: 4.5 Mile Run + Strength

Warm Up
1 Minute of walking
3 Minutes of jogging at a slow pace
Mobility drills (high knees, heel flicks, hip circles)
17 side lying leg raises (each side)
17 glute bridges
1 Minute of jogging at a slow pace

Briefing: Complete a 4 Mile run at a steady pace followed by a strength circuit: Squats x 27 Press ups x 17 Single Leg Romanian Dead lifts x 17 (each side) Plank 60 seconds Body Row x 19	Stretches:
Time:	Target for next session:

Notes: use this area to write any notes related to performance, session, how you are feeling etc

Sleep		
What time you went to bed:	What time you woke up:	Total hours sleep:

Day 39: Walk

Briefing: Complete a 60-90 minute walk 16 side lying leg raises (each side) 16 glute bridges	Stretches:

Notes: use this area to write any notes related to performance, session, how you are feeling etc

Sleep		
What time you went to bed:	What time you woke up:	Total hours sleep:

Day 40: 4.5 Mile Run

Warm Up
1 Minute of walking
3 Minutes of jogging at a slow pace
Mobility drills (high knees, heel flicks, hip circles)
17 side lying leg raises (each side)
17 glute bridges
1 Minute of jogging at a slow pace

Briefing: Complete a 4.5 Mile run at a steady pace	Stretches:
Time:	Target for next session:
Notes:	

Sleep		
What time you went to bed:	What time you woke up:	Total hours sleep:

Day 41: Strength

Warm Up
1 Minute of walking
3 Minutes of jogging at a slow pace
Mobility drills (high knees, heel flicks, hip circles)
17 side lying leg raises (each side)
17 glute bridges
1 Minute of jogging at a slow pace
Alternatively, you can use a cross trainer or a rower to warm up for 5 minutes, but still perform the mobility drills and activation exercises

Briefing: Complete 2 rounds of the circuit	Stretches:
Squats x 27	
Press ups x 18	
Single Leg Romanian Dead lifts x 17 (each side)	
Plank 60 seconds	
Body Row x 19	
Time:	Target for next session:
Notes:	

Sleep		
What time you went to bed:	What time you woke up:	Total hours sleep:

Day 42: Rest

Briefing: Rest and relax. Do not do anything intense on this day. Gentle walk, swimming, mobility drills are OK and recommended.

Notes: *Reflect on the progress you have made this week.*

Sleep

What time you went to bed:	What time you woke up:	Total hours sleep:

Test Week Schedule

Day / Week	1	2	3	4	5	6	7
1	Rest	1.5 Mile Run Test	Walk	3 Mile Run Slow + Strength	Walk	Strength	Rest

Once you have completed the test take the rest of this week as active recovery before beginning the Recruit Training Programme. This is a de-load week and it is to allow your body to recover and to promote the necessary adaptations to occur.

Day 1: Rest

Briefing: Rest and relax. Do not do anything intense on this day. Gentle walk, swimming, mobility drills are OK and recommended.

Notes: *Visualise your success in tomorrow's test.*

Sleep

What time you went to bed:	What time you woke up:	Total hours sleep:

Day 2: Test

Take 2 days of rest and then undertake 1.5 mile run test again. Ensure it is in the same conditions as the first test 6 weeks ago. For example; if you conducted the test on a treadmill the first time, perform this test on a treadmill.
Spend 15 minutes warming up and then run 1.5 miles as quick as you can. This test is ideally performed on a running track; however, a treadmill can be used (1% gradient must be applied).

Rating	Time
Poor	>16:01
Fair	16:00-12:01
Good	12:00-10:31
Excellent	10:30-09:30
Superior	<09:29

Use the score sheet to make a log of your scores (the extra boxes are to allow you to use this programme multiple times if you wish to)

Date				
Your Time				
Target for next test				

Briefing: After test rest and relax. Do not do anything intense on this day. Gentle walk, swimming, mobility drills are OK and recommended.

Sleep		
What time you went to bed:	What time you woke up:	Total hours sleep:

Day 3: Walk

Briefing: Complete a 60-90 minute walk 17 side lying leg raises (each side) 17 glute bridges	Stretches:

Notes:

Sleep		
What time you went to bed:	What time you woke up:	Total hours sleep:

Day 4: 3 Mile Run + Strength

Warm Up
1 Minute of walking
3 Minutes of jogging at a slow pace
Mobility drills (high knees, heel flicks, hip circles)
17 side lying leg raises (each side)
17 glute bridges
1 Minute of jogging at a slow pace

Briefing: Complete a 3 Mile run at a slow pace followed by a strength circuit: Squats x 25 Press ups x 15 Single Leg Romanian Dead lifts x 15 (each side) Plank 60 seconds Body Row x 17	Stretches:

Notes: use this area to write any notes related to performance, session, how you are feeling etc

There is no requirement to time this run or circuit, relax.

Sleep		
What time you went to bed:	What time you woke up:	Total hours sleep:

Day 5: Walk

Briefing: Complete a 60-90 minute walk 18 side lying leg raises (each side) 18 glute bridges	Stretches:

Notes: use this area to write any notes related to performance, session, how you are feeling etc

Sleep		
What time you went to bed:	What time you woke up:	Total hours sleep:

Day 6: Strength

Warm Up
1 Minute of walking
3 Minutes of jogging at a slow pace
Mobility drills (high knees, heel flicks, hip circles)
17 side lying leg raises (each side)
17 glute bridges
1 Minute of jogging at a slow pace
Alternatively, you can use a cross trainer or a rower to warm up for 5 minutes, but still perform the mobility drills and activation exercises

Briefing: Complete 2 rounds of the circuit Squats x 25 Press ups x 16 Single Leg Romanian Dead lifts x 15 (each side) Plank 60 seconds Body Row x 17	Stretches:

Notes: *use this area to write any notes related to performance, session, how you are feeling etc*

There is no requirement to time this circuit, relax.

Sleep

What time you went to bed:	What time you woke up:	Total hours sleep:

Day 7: Rest

Briefing: Rest and relax. Do not do anything intense on this day. Gentle walk, swimming, mobility drills are OK and recommended.

Notes:

Sleep

What time you went to bed:	What time you woke up:	Total hours sleep:

Recruit Training Programme Schedule

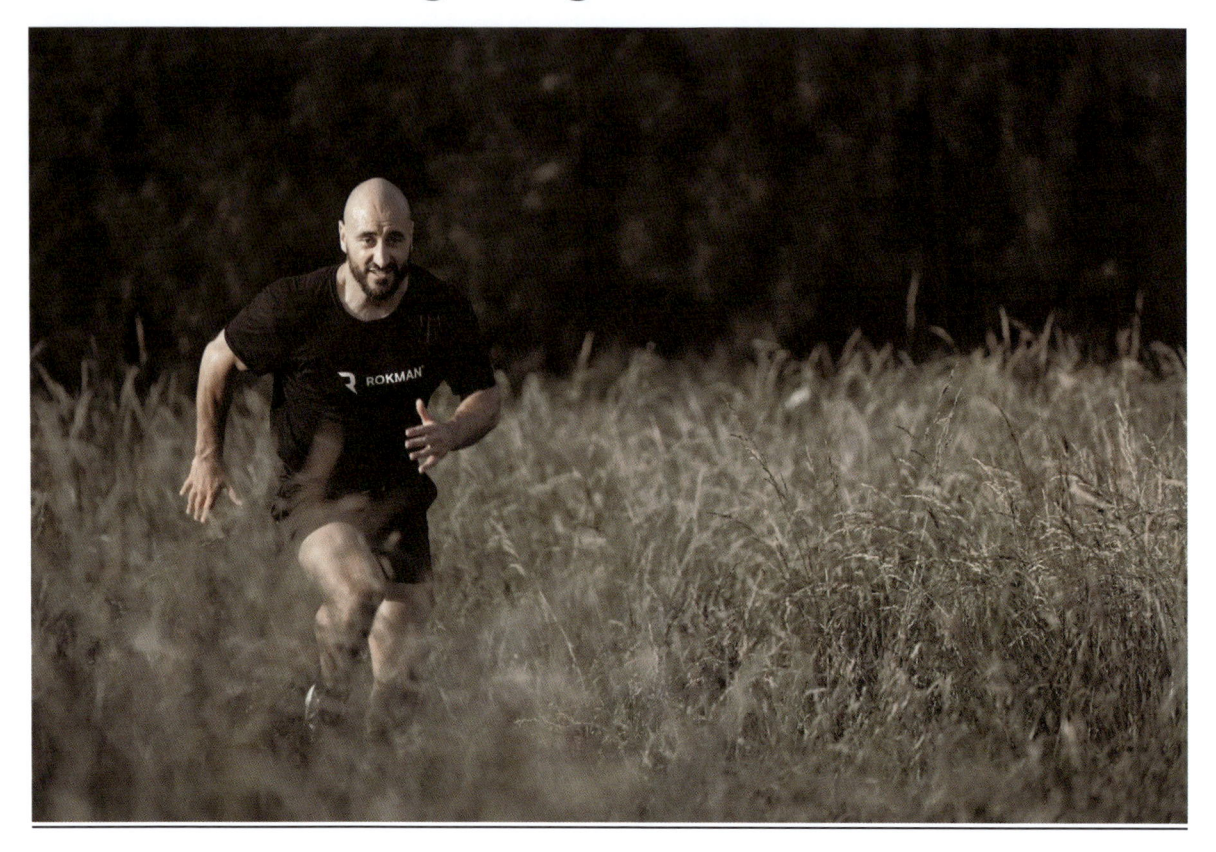

Day / Week	1	2	3	4	5	6	7
1	5 Mile Run Steady	Walk	Hill Sprints + Strength	Walk	4 Mile Run Moderate	Strength	Rest
2	5.5 Mile Run Steady	Walk	Hill Sprints + Strength	Walk	4 Mile Run Moderate	Strength	Rest
3	6 Mile Run Steady	Walk	Hill Sprints + Strength	Walk	4 Mile Run Moderate	Strength	Rest
4	6.5 Mile Run Steady	Walk	Hill Sprints + Strength	Walk	800m Sprints	Strength	Rest
5	7 Mile Run	Walk	Hill Sprints + Strength	Walk	800m Sprints	Strength	Rest
6	7.5 Mile Run	Walk	Hill Sprints + Strength	Walk	800m Sprints	Strength	Rest

Day 1: 5 Mile Run

Warm Up
1 Minute of walking
3 Minutes of jogging at a slow pace
Mobility drills (high knees, heel flicks, hip circles)
18 side lying leg raises (each side)
18 glute bridges
1 Minute of jogging at a slow pace

Briefing: Complete a 5 Mile run at a steady pace	Stretches:
Time:	Target for next session:

Notes: *use this area to write any notes related to performance, session, how you are feeling etc*

Sleep		
What time you went to bed:	What time you woke up:	Total hours sleep:

Day 2: Walk

Briefing: Complete a 60-90 minute walk 18 side lying leg raises (each side) 18 glute bridges	Stretches:

Notes: *use this area to write any notes related to performance, session, how you are feeling etc*

Sleep		
What time you went to bed:	What time you woke up:	Total hours sleep:

Day 3: Hill Sprints + Strength

Warm Up
1 Minute of walking
3 Minutes of jogging at a slow pace
Mobility drills (high knees, heel flicks, hip circles)
18 side lying leg raises (each side)
18 glute bridges
1 Minute of jogging at a slow pace

Briefing: Complete a series of 3 maximum effort hill sprints followed by Squats x 26 Press ups x 16 Single Leg Romanian Dead lifts x 16 (each side) Plank 60 seconds Body Row x 18	Stretches:
Circuit Time:	Target for next session:

Notes: *use this area to write any notes related to performance, session, how you are feeling etc*

Sleep		
What time you went to bed:	What time you woke up:	Total hours sleep:

Day 4: Walk

Briefing: Complete a 60-90 minute walk 18 side lying leg raises (each side) 18 glute bridges	Stretches:

Notes: *use this area to write any notes related to performance, session, how you are feeling etc*

Sleep		
What time you went to bed:	What time you woke up:	Total hours sleep:

Day 5: 4 Mile Run

Warm Up	
1 Minute of walking 3 Minutes of jogging at a slow pace Mobility drills (high knees, heel flicks, hip circles) 19 side lying leg raises (each side) 19 glute bridges 1 Minute of jogging at a slow pace	
Briefing: Complete a 4 Mile run at a **moderate pace**	Stretches:
Time:	Target for next session:
Notes:	
Sleep	
What time you went to bed:	What time you woke up:	Total hours sleep:

Day 6: Strength

Warm Up	
1 Minute of walking 3 Minutes of jogging at a slow pace Mobility drills (high knees, heel flicks, hip circles) 20 side lying leg raises (each side) 20 glute bridges 1 Minute of jogging at a slow pace *Alternatively, you can use a cross trainer or a rower to warm up for 5 minutes, but still perform the mobility drills and activation exercises*	
Briefing: Complete 2 rounds of the circuit Weighted Squats x 10 Press ups x 18 Weighted Single Leg Romanian Dead lifts x 10 (each side) Burpee x 10 Body Row x 20	Stretches:
Time:	Target for next session:
Notes:	
Weight used for Squats:	
Weight used for SLRDL:	
Sleep	
What time you went to bed:	What time you woke up:	Total hours sleep:

Day 7: Rest

Briefing: Rest and relax. Do not do anything intense on this day. Gentle walk, swimming, mobility drills, yoga or sports massage are recommended.

Notes: Reflect on the progress you have made this week. Think about what you are going to achieve over the next week.

Sleep

What time you went to bed:	What time you woke up:	Total hours sleep:

Day 8: 5.5 Mile Run

Warm Up
1 Minute of walking
3 Minutes of jogging at a slow pace
Mobility drills (high knees, heel flicks, hip circles)
20 side lying leg raises (each side)
20 glute bridges
1 Minute of jogging at a slow pace

Briefing: Complete a 5.5 Mile run at a steady pace	**Stretches:**
Time:	**Target for next session:**

Notes: use this area to write any notes related to performance, session, how you are feeling etc

Sleep

What time you went to bed:	What time you woke up:	Total hours sleep:

Day 9: Walk

Briefing: Complete a 60-90 minute walk 20 side lying leg raises (each side) 20 glute bridges	Stretches:
Notes: use this area to write any notes related to performance, session, how you are feeling etc	
Sleep	
What time you went to bed:	What time you woke up:	Total hours sleep:

Day 10: Hill Sprints + Strength

Warm Up 1 Minute of walking 3 Minutes of jogging at a slow pace Mobility drills (high knees, heel flicks, hip circles) 21 side lying leg raises (each side) 21 glute bridges 1 Minute of jogging at a slow pace	
Briefing: Complete a series of 4 maximum effort hill sprints followed by: Squats x 27 Press ups x 17 Single Leg Romanian Dead lifts x 17 (each side) Plank 60 seconds Body Row x 20	Stretches:
Circuit Time:	Target for next session:
Notes: use this area to write any notes related to performance, session, how you are feeling etc	
Sleep	
What time you went to bed:	What time you woke up:	Total hours sleep:

Day 11: Walk

Briefing: Complete a 60-90 minute walk 21 side lying leg raises (each side) 21 glute bridges	Stretches:
Notes: *use this area to write any notes related to performance, session, how you are feeling etc*	
Sleep	
What time you went to bed:	What time you woke up:	Total hours sleep:

Day 12: 4 Mile Run

Warm Up
1 Minute of walking
3 Minutes of jogging at a slow pace
Mobility drills (high knees, heel flicks, hip circles)
21 side lying leg raises (each side)
21 glute bridges
1 Minute of jogging at a slow pace

Briefing: Complete a 4 Mile run at a moderate pace	Stretches:
Time:	Target for next session:
Notes: *use this area to write any notes related to performance, session, how you are feeling etc*	
Sleep	
What time you went to bed:	What time you woke up:	Total hours sleep:

Day 13: Strength

Warm Up
1 Minute of walking
3 Minutes of jogging at a slow pace
Mobility drills (high knees, heel flicks, hip circles)
22 side lying leg raises (each side)
22 glute bridges
1 Minute of jogging at a slow pace
Alternatively, you can use a cross trainer or a rower to warm up for 5 minutes, but still perform the mobility drills and activation exercises

Briefing: Complete 2 rounds of the circuit Weighted Squats x 10 Press ups x 18 Weighted Single Leg Romanian Dead lifts x 10 (each side) Burpee x 10 Body Row x 20	Stretches:
Time:	Target for next session:

Notes: *use this area to write any notes related to performance, session, how you are feeling etc*

Weights used for squats:
Weights used for SLRDL:
(Aim to increase by 2.5kg, as long as you maintain good form)

Sleep		
What time you went to bed:	What time you woke up:	Total hours sleep:

Day 14: Rest

Briefing: Rest and relax. Do not do anything intense on this day. Gentle walk, swimming, mobility drills, yoga or sports massage are recommended.

Notes: *Reflect on the progress you have made this week. Think about what you are going to achieve over the next week.*

Sleep		
What time you went to bed:	What time you woke up:	Total hours sleep:

Day 15: 6 Mile Run

Warm Up
1 Minute of walking
3 Minutes of jogging at a slow pace
Mobility drills (high knees, heel flicks, hip circles)
22 side lying leg raises (each side)
22 glute bridges
1 Minute of jogging at a slow pace

Briefing: Complete a 6 Mile run at a steady pace	**Stretches:**
Time:	**Target for next session:**

Notes: use this area to write any notes related to performance, session, how you are feeling etc

Sleep

What time you went to bed:	What time you woke up:	Total hours sleep:

Day 16: Walk

Briefing: Complete a 60-90 minute walk 22 side lying leg raises (each side) 22 glute bridges	**Stretches:**

Notes: use this area to write any notes related to performance, session, how you are feeling etc

Sleep

What time you went to bed:	What time you woke up:	Total hours sleep:

Day 17: Hill Sprints + Strength

Warm Up
1 Minute of walking
3 Minutes of jogging at a slow pace
Mobility drills (high knees, heel flicks, hip circles)
23 side lying leg raises (each side)
23 glute bridges
1 Minute of jogging at a slow pace

Briefing: Complete a series of 5 maximum effort hill sprints followed by: Squats x 27 Press ups x 17 Single Leg Romanian Dead lifts x 17 (each side) Plank 60 seconds Body Row x 20	Stretches:
Circuit Time:	**Target for next session:**

Notes: *use this area to write any notes related to performance, session, how you are feeling etc*

Sleep		
What time you went to bed:	What time you woke up:	Total hours sleep:

Day 18: Walk

Briefing: Complete a 60-90 minute walk 23 side lying leg raises (each side) 23 glute bridges	Stretches:

Notes: *use this area to write any notes related to performance, session, how you are feeling etc*

Sleep		
What time you went to bed:	What time you woke up:	Total hours sleep:

Day 19: 4 Mile Run

Warm Up		
1 Minute of walking 3 Minutes of jogging at a slow pace Mobility drills (high knees, heel flicks, hip circles) 23 side lying leg raises (each side) 23 glute bridges 1 Minute of jogging at a slow pace		
Briefing: Complete a 4 Mile run at a **moderate pace**		**Stretches:**
Time:		**Target for next session:**
Notes:		
Sleep		
What time you went to bed:	What time you woke up:	Total hours sleep:

Day 20: Strength

Warm Up		
1 Minute of walking 3 Minutes of jogging at a slow pace Mobility drills (high knees, heel flicks, hip circles) 23 side lying leg raises (each side) 23 glute bridges 1 Minute of jogging at a slow pace *Alternatively, you can use a cross trainer or a rower to warm up for 5 minutes, but still perform the mobility drills and activation exercises*		
Briefing: Complete 2 rounds of the circuit Weighted Squats x 10 Press ups x 19 Weighted Single Leg Romanian Dead lifts x 10 (each side) Burpee x 10 Body Row x 20		**Stretches:**
Time:		
Notes:		
Weights used for squats:		
Weights used for SLRDL:		
(Aim to increase by 2.5kg, as long as you maintain good form)		
Sleep		
What time you went to bed:	What time you woke up:	Total hours sleep:

Day 21: Rest

Briefing: Rest and relax. Do not do anything intense on this day. Gentle walk, swimming, mobility drills, yoga or sports massage are recommended.
Notes: *Reflect on the progress you have made this week. Think about what you are going to achieve over the next week.*

Sleep		
What time you went to bed:	What time you woke up:	Total hours sleep:

Day 22: 6.5 Mile Run

Warm Up
1 Minute of walking
3 Minutes of jogging at a slow pace
Mobility drills (high knees, heel flicks, hip circles)
23 side lying leg raises (each side)
23 glute bridges
1 Minute of jogging at a slow pace

Briefing: Complete a 6.5 Mile run at a steady pace	Stretches:
Time:	Target for next session:
Notes: *use this area to write any notes related to performance, session, how you are feeling etc*	

Sleep		
What time you went to bed:	What time you woke up:	Total hours sleep:

Day 23: Walk

Briefing: Complete a 60-90 minute walk 24 side lying leg raises (each side) 24 glute bridges	Stretches:
Notes: use this area to write any notes related to performance, session, how you are feeling etc	

Sleep		
What time you went to bed:	What time you woke up:	Total hours sleep:

Day 24: Hill Sprints + Strength

Warm Up 1 Minute of walking 3 Minutes of jogging at a slow pace Mobility drills (high knees, heel flicks, hip circles) 24 side lying leg raises (each side) 24 glute bridges 1 Minute of jogging at a slow pace	
Briefing: Complete a series of 6 maximum effort hill sprints followed by: Squats x 27 Press ups x 17 Single Leg Romanian Dead lifts x 17 (each side) Plank 60 seconds Body Row x 20	Stretches:
Circuit Time:	**Target for next session:**
Notes: use this area to write any notes related to performance, session, how you are feeling etc	

Sleep		
What time you went to bed:	What time you woke up:	Total hours sleep:

Day 25: Walk

Briefing: Complete a 60-90 minute walk 24 side lying leg raises (each side) 24 glute bridges	Stretches:
Notes:	

Sleep		
What time you went to bed:	What time you woke up:	Total hours sleep:

Day 26: 800m Sprints

Warm Up 1 Minute of walking 5 Minutes of jogging at a slow pace Mobility drills (high knees, heel flicks, hip circles) 24 side lying leg raises (each side) 24 glute bridges 2 Minutes of jogging at a slow pace Run 100metres at 85% effort 2 minutes jogging at slow pace Run 100metres at 90% effort 2 minutes jogging at slow pace 30 seconds rest before starting the sprint	
Briefing: Perform 2 x **800 metre** sprint 100% effort. Rest for 2 minutes between each sprint (do not allow yourself to get cold). **Scores** | Cook	3:15
Infantry	2:46 – 3:15
Commando	Less than 2:45		Stretches:

Sprint 1 time:	Target for next session:
Sprint 2 time:	Target for next session:
Notes:	

Sleep		
What time you went to bed:	What time you woke up:	Total hours sleep:

Day 27: Strength

Warm Up
1 Minute of walking
3 Minutes of jogging at a slow pace
Mobility drills (high knees, heel flicks, hip circles)
24 side lying leg raises (each side)
24 glute bridges
1 Minute of jogging at a slow pace
Alternatively, you can use a cross trainer or a rower to warm up for 5 minutes, but still perform the mobility drills and activation exercises

Briefing: Complete 3 rounds of the circuit	Stretches:
Weighted Squats x 10	
Jump squats (bodyweight only) x 10	
Press ups x 20	
Weighted Single Leg Romanian Dead lifts x 10 (each side)	
Burpee x 10	
Body Row x 20	
Time:	**Target for next session:**

Notes: *use this area to write any notes related to performance, session, how you are feeling etc*

Weights used for squats:

Weights used for SLRDL:

(Aim to increase by 2.5kg, as long as you maintain good form)

Sleep

What time you went to bed:	What time you woke up:	Total hours sleep:

Day 28: Rest

Briefing: Rest and relax. Do not do anything intense on this day. Gentle walk, swimming, mobility drills, yoga or sports massage are recommended.

Notes: *Reflect on the progress you have made this week. Think about what you are going to achieve over the next week.*

Sleep

What time you went to bed:	What time you woke up:	Total hours sleep:

Day 29: 7 Mile Run

Warm Up
1 Minute of walking
3 Minutes of jogging at a slow pace
Mobility drills (high knees, heel flicks, hip circles)
25 side lying leg raises (each side)
25 glute bridges
1 Minute of jogging at a slow pace

Briefing: Complete a 7 Mile run at a steady pace	Stretches:
Time:	Target for next session:
Notes: use this area to write any notes related to performance, session, how you are feeling etc	
Sleep	
What time you went to bed:	What time you woke up:	Total hours sleep:

Day 30: Walk

Briefing: Complete a 60-90 minute walk	Stretches:
25 side lying leg raises (each side)	
25 glute bridges	
Notes: use this area to write any notes related to performance, session, how you are feeling etc	
Sleep	
What time you went to bed:	What time you woke up:	Total hours sleep:

Day 31: Hill Sprints + Strength

Warm Up
1 Minute of walking
3 Minutes of jogging at a slow pace
Mobility drills (high knees, heel flicks, hip circles)
25 side lying leg raises (each side)
25 glute bridges
1 Minute of jogging at a slow pace

Briefing: Complete a series of 7 maximum effort hill sprints followed by: Squats x 27 Press ups x 17 Single Leg Romanian Dead lifts x 17 (each side) Plank 60 seconds Body Row x 20	Stretches:
Circuit Time:	**Target for next session:**

Notes: *use this area to write any notes related to performance, session, how you are feeling etc*

Sleep		
What time you went to bed:	What time you woke up:	Total hours sleep:

Day 32: Walk

Briefing: Complete a 60-90 minute walk 25 side lying leg raises (each side) 25 glute bridges	Stretches:

Notes: *use this area to write any notes related to performance, session, how you are feeling etc*

Sleep		
What time you went to bed:	What time you woke up:	Total hours sleep:

Day 33: 800 Metre Sprints

Warm Up
1 Minute of walking
5 Minutes of jogging at a slow pace
Mobility drills (high knees, heel flicks, hip circles)
25 side lying leg raises (each side)
25 glute bridges
2 Minutes of jogging at a slow pace
Run 100metres at 85% effort
2 minutes jogging at slow pace
Run 100metres at 90% effort
2 minutes jogging at slow pace
30 seconds rest before starting the sprint

Briefing: Perform 2 x **800 metre** sprint 100% effort. Rest for 2 minutes between each sprint (do not allow yourself to get cold).

Stretches:

Scores

Cook	3:15
Infantry	2:46 – 3:15
Commando	Less than 2:45

Sprint 1 time:

Target for next session:

Sprint 2 time:

Target for next session:

Notes: use this area to write any notes related to performance, session, how you are feeling etc

Sleep

| What time you went to bed: | What time you woke up: | Total hours sleep: |

Day 34: Strength

Warm Up
1 Minute of walking
3 Minutes of jogging at a slow pace
Mobility drills (high knees, heel flicks, hip circles)
26 side lying leg raises (each side)
26 glute bridges
1 Minute of jogging at a slow pace
Alternatively, you can use a cross trainer or a rower to warm up for 5 minutes, but still perform the mobility drills and activation exercises

Briefing: Complete 3 rounds of the circuit	Stretches:
Weighted Squats x 10	
Jump Squats (bodyweight only) x 10	
Press ups x 20	
Weighted Single Leg Romanian Dead lifts x 10 (each side)	
Burpee x 10	
Body Row x 20	
Time:	**Target for next session:**

Notes: *use this area to write any notes related to performance, session, how you are feeling etc*

Weights used for squats:

Weights used for SLRDL:

(Aim to increase by 2.5kg, as long as you maintain good form)

Sleep		
What time you went to bed:	What time you woke up:	Total hours sleep:

Day 35: Rest

Briefing: Rest and relax. Do not do anything intense on this day. Gentle walk, swimming, mobility drills, yoga or sports massage are recommended.

Notes: *Reflect on the progress you have made this week. Think about what you are going to achieve over the next week.*

Sleep		
What time you went to bed:	What time you woke up:	Total hours sleep:

Day 36: 7.5 Mile Run

Warm Up
1 Minute of walking
3 Minutes of jogging at a slow pace
Mobility drills (high knees, heel flicks, hip circles)
26 side lying leg raises (each side)
26 glute bridges
1 Minute of jogging at a slow pace

Briefing: Complete a 7.5 Mile run at a steady pace	Stretches:
Time:	Target for next session:

Notes: *use this area to write any notes related to performance, session, how you are feeling etc*

Sleep		
What time you went to bed:	What time you woke up:	Total hours sleep:

Day 37: Walk

Briefing: Complete a 60-90 minute walk 26 side lying leg raises (each side) 26 glute bridges	Stretches:

Notes: *use this area to write any notes related to performance, session, how you are feeling etc*

Sleep		
What time you went to bed:	What time you woke up:	Total hours sleep:

Day 38: Hill Sprints + Strength

Warm Up
1 Minute of walking
3 Minutes of jogging at a slow pace
Mobility drills (high knees, heel flicks, hip circles)
27 side lying leg raises (each side)
27 glute bridges
1 Minute of jogging at a slow pace

Briefing: Complete a series of 8 maximum effort hill sprints followed by: Squats x 27 Press ups x 17 Single Leg Romanian Dead lifts x 17 (each side) Plank 60 seconds Body Row x 20	Stretches:
Circuit Time:	Target for next session:

Notes: use this area to write any notes related to performance, session, how you are feeling etc

Sleep		
What time you went to bed:	What time you woke up:	Total hours sleep:

Day 39: Walk

Briefing: Complete a 60-90 minute walk 27 side lying leg raises (each side) 27 glute bridges	Stretches:

Notes: use this area to write any notes related to performance, session, how you are feeling etc

Sleep		
What time you went to bed:	What time you woke up:	Total hours sleep:

Day 40: 800 metre sprints

Warm Up
1 Minute of walking
5 Minutes of jogging at a slow pace
Mobility drills (high knees, heel flicks, hip circles)
27 side lying leg raises (each side)
27 glute bridges
2 Minutes of jogging at a slow pace
Run 100metres at 85% effort
2 minutes jogging at slow pace
Run 100metres at 90% effort
2 minutes jogging at slow pace
30 seconds rest before starting the sprint

Briefing: Perform **3 x 800 metre** sprints 100% effort. Rest for 2 minutes between each sprint (do not allow yourself to get cold).

Scores

Cook	3:15
Infantry	2:46 – 3:15
Commando	Less than 2:45

Stretches:

Sprint 1 time:

Sprint 2 time:

Sprint 3 time:

Notes: use this area to write any notes related to performance, session, how you are feeling etc

Sleep		
What time you went to bed:	What time you woke up:	Total hours sleep:

Day 41: Strength

Warm Up
1 Minute of walking
3 Minutes of jogging at a slow pace
Mobility drills (high knees, heel flicks, hip circles)
28 side lying leg raises (each side)
28 glute bridges
1 Minute of jogging at a slow pace
Alternatively, you can use a cross trainer or a rower to warm up for 5 minutes, but still perform the mobility drills and activation exercises

Briefing: Complete 3 rounds of the circuit Weighted Squats x 10 Jump Squats (bodyweight only) x 10 Press ups x 20 Weighted Single Leg Romanian Dead lifts x 10 (each side) Burpee x 10 Body Row x 20	**Stretches:**
Time:	**Target for next session:**

Notes: *use this area to write any notes related to performance, session, how you are feeling etc*

Weights used for squats:
Weights used for SLRDL:
(Aim to increase by 2.5kg, as long as you maintain good form)

Sleep		
What time you went to bed:	What time you woke up:	Total hours sleep:

Day 42: Rest

Briefing: Rest and relax. Do not do anything intense on this day. Gentle walk, swimming, mobility drills, yoga or sports massage are recommended.

Notes: *Reflect on the progress you have made this week. Think about what you are going to achieve over the next week.*

Sleep		
What time you went to bed:	What time you woke up:	Total hours sleep:

Day 43: Rest

Briefing: Rest and relax. Do not do anything intense on this day. Gentle walk, swimming, mobility drills are OK and recommended.

Notes: Visualise your success in tomorrow's test.

Sleep

What time you went to bed:	What time you woke up:	Total hours sleep:

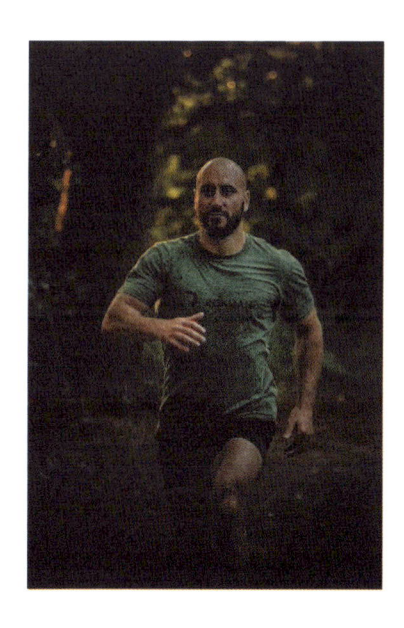

GET READY FOR TEST DAY!

Day 44: Test

After 2 days of rest undertake the 1.5 mile run test again. Ensure it is in the same conditions as the first test 6 weeks ago. For example; if you conducted the test on a treadmill the first time, perform this test on a treadmill. Spend 15 minutes warming up and then run 1.5 miles as quick as you can. This test is ideally performed on a running track; however, a treadmill can be used (1% gradient must be applied).

Rating	Time
Poor	>16:01
Fair	16:00-12:01
Good	12:00-10:31
Excellent	10:30-09:30
Superior	<09:29

Use the score sheet to make a log of your scores (the extra boxes are to allow you to use this programme multiple times if you wish to)

Date				
Your Time				

Briefing: After test rest and relax. Do not do anything intense on this day. Gentle walk, swimming, mobility drills are OK and recommended.

Sleep		
What time you went to bed:	What time you woke up:	Total hours sleep:

Beyond Commando Runner

Congratulations! You have just completed the training programme. You should have made a noticeable improvement in your 1.5 mile run time and be running faster and feel fitter and stronger.

What you do next is entirely up to you. I would recommend taking a week of active recovery where you reduce your running and intensity.

It could be time for you to build your own running programme or you could repeat the Commando Runner programme and make your own tweaks.

Here are some considerations if you are looking to design your own programme.

- Focus on consistency – many trainees burn themselves out by starting off with a real intense programme that they simply cannot maintain
- Progression – The mileage and intensity should gradually build up over time so that your body can adapt
- Plan – It is a good idea to plan your training schedule so that your intense / high impact days are spread out. This will enable you to recover and perform better whilst reducing the likelihood of injury
- Rest – An often overlooked part of the programme. Sometimes less is more, as you can make your sessions more intense and recover better from them

When I was a teenager training to get fit for the Royal Marines, I was so keen that I trained three times a day! My routine looked a bit like this:

1. Morning Run
2. Afternoon Circuit Training (with bodyweight and sprints)
3. Evening Circuit training (with light weights)

Sometimes I would do sprints in the evening circuit training session too. Looking at this programme now I realise that there is too much running. I was running three times a day!

The result of this was that I ended up with shin splints before I even went to the Royal Marines selection course. After I completed the Potential Royal Marines Course, I continued training even harder than I had before and my shin splints got worse. I then began Recruit Training and spent most of the 33 weeks of training in agony as my shin splints turned into stress fractures.

All of this could have been avoided if I had planned my training better. Royal Marines training is notoriously difficult and I made it even harder for myself by going in with an injury.

With your current level of fitness, you should be able to go out and find a lot of enjoyment in runs. Here are some running challenges you may want to try.

Running Pyramid

For this you will need a timer, and some way of measuring distance such as a GPS tracker. As always ensure you warm up adequately prior to starting.

Run as far as you can for 5 minutes
Rest 60 seconds
Run as far as you can for 4 minutes
Rest 60 seconds
Ru as far as you can for 3 minutes

Make a note of your distances and try and beat them as your fitness improves.

The Mile Run

This is a simple one but can be quite brutal. After a thorough warm up, you simply run 1 mile as fast as you can.

Fun Fact! The World Record is currently **3:43:13**, set by Hicham El Guerrouj of Morocco in 1999.

Negative Splits

When running, usually we start off quicker and the longer we run for the slower we get as we are fatigued. The negative split challenge changes that. The aim is to run each mile (or whatever interval split you choose) quicker each time.

Pick whatever distance you want, a successful negative split for a 5 mile run for someone with an average split pace of 7:15 would look something like this:

Mile 1 7:15
Mile 2 7:10
Mile 3 7:03
Mile 4 7:00
Mile 5 6:49

This isn't an excuse to start off slow and gradually get quicker by the way as this is a challenge! The aim is to increase your fitness, endurance and mental toughness.

==If you are going to be completing the Commando Runner programme again, you could replace the moderate pace run with a negative split run.==

Run a Marathon

Perhaps the most synonymous "race" when it comes to running. You can either enter an event or have a go doing the distance yourself. The marathon is 26.2 miles which is quite a challenging distance.

A way of making a marathon fun if you have a training partner is taking it in turns to do a mile each. So, you end up doing a half marathon each in intervals. Due to the amount of rest you are able to get the pace for 1 mile intervals can be quite fast.

Want to make it even more challenging? Combine this partner challenge with the negative splits challenge! Remember the faster you go, the less rest your partner has! This is a tough one by the way!

Bleep Test Circuit

On the subject of partner workouts this is best done with a partner but can also be done solo.

You will need a 20 metre long area for sprints such as a sports hall. You will also need an audio of the 20 metre bleep test.

After a thorough warm up, you run 3 bleeps, then perform exercises for 3 bleeps. Exercises such as listed below usually work pretty well:

- Press ups
- Squats
- Burpees
- Sit ups

Alternate with your partner so when you're doing the exercises they are running. Feel free to add whatever exercises you want to make this one more challenging. Try and keep up with the beep. The break from running should allow you to keep up with it for a lot longer than normal.

Alternative Exercises

You may need this section if:

- You have completed the Commando Runner Programme and are attempting it again and wanted to use some different exercises within the circuit
- You are unable to do the exercises listed in the circuit for whatever reasons

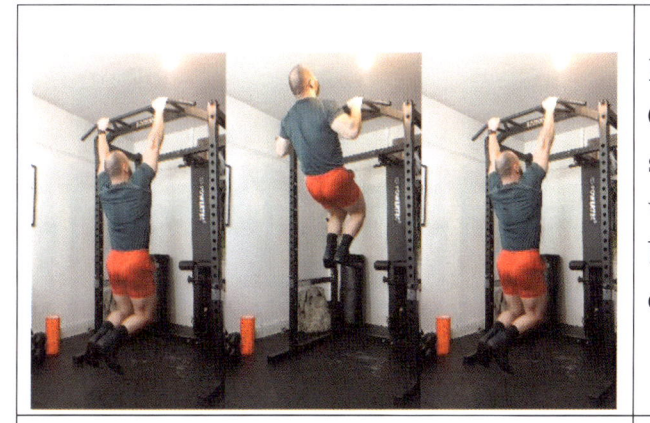

Pull Ups *(instead, or along with body row)*
Grab the bar with an overhand grip with hands slightly wider than shoulder width apart. Hang with your feet off the floor. Pull your chest to the bar and slowly lower down until arms are fully extended.

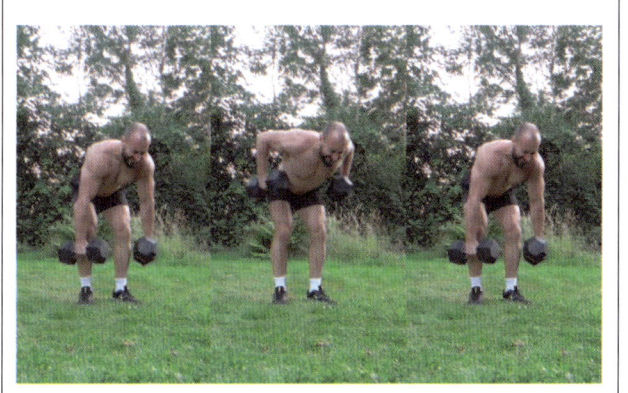

Bent Over Row *(instead of body row)*
(pictured with dumbbells, can be performed with a barbell)
Grip the (barbell) with an overhand grip, drive up using your legs. Stand tall, then push your hips back and bend your knees slightly keeping your chest out.
Row the elbows backwards, bringing the bar towards your stomach. Slowly lower down.

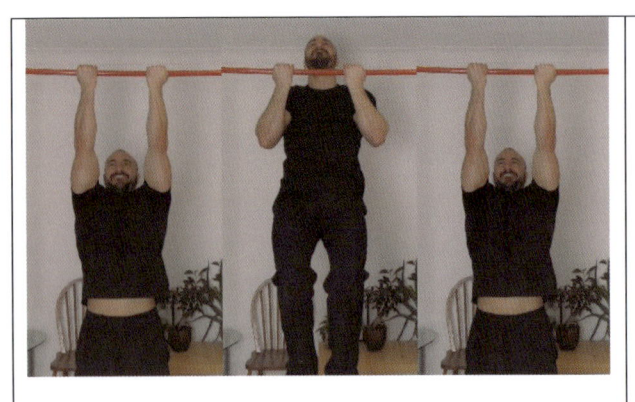

Chin Ups *(instead, or along with body row)*
Grip hold of the bar with palms slightly narrower than shoulder width apart, palms facing towards you.
Pull yourself up until your chin is over the bar and slowly lower yourself down until arms are extended.

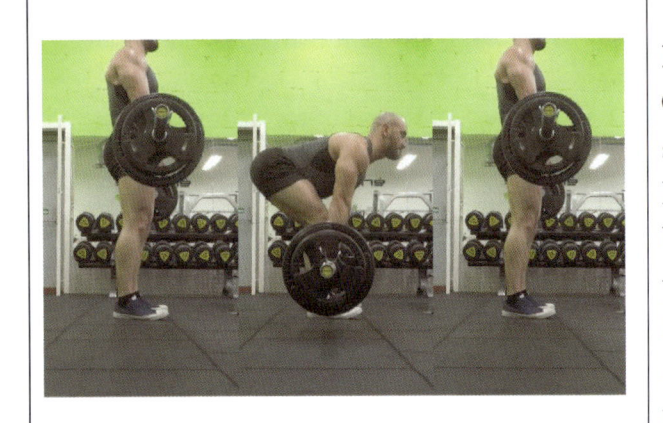

Romanian Deadlift *(instead of single leg RDL)*
Grip the bar with an overhand grip, feet about shoulder width apart toes pointing forwards. From the standing position, push your hips back and bend your knees slightly, keeping your chest out. Go until you feel a stretch on the hamstring and then extend back up to the starting position. Keep the bar close to your body.

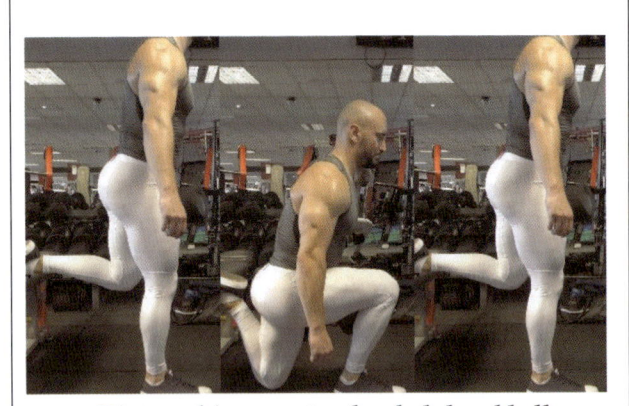

Pictured is a contra-loaded dumbbell

Bulgarian Split Squat *(instead of squats)*
With rear foot elevated, knees tracking the toe, slowly lower yourself down until the kneel is just touching the floor and then drive up with the front leg.
- Beginner version - bodyweight only
- Progression - hold a dumbbell on the side of the working leg, gradually increase weight over time
- Advanced version – Hold a dumbbell on the opposite side to the working leg (pictured)

Author Profile

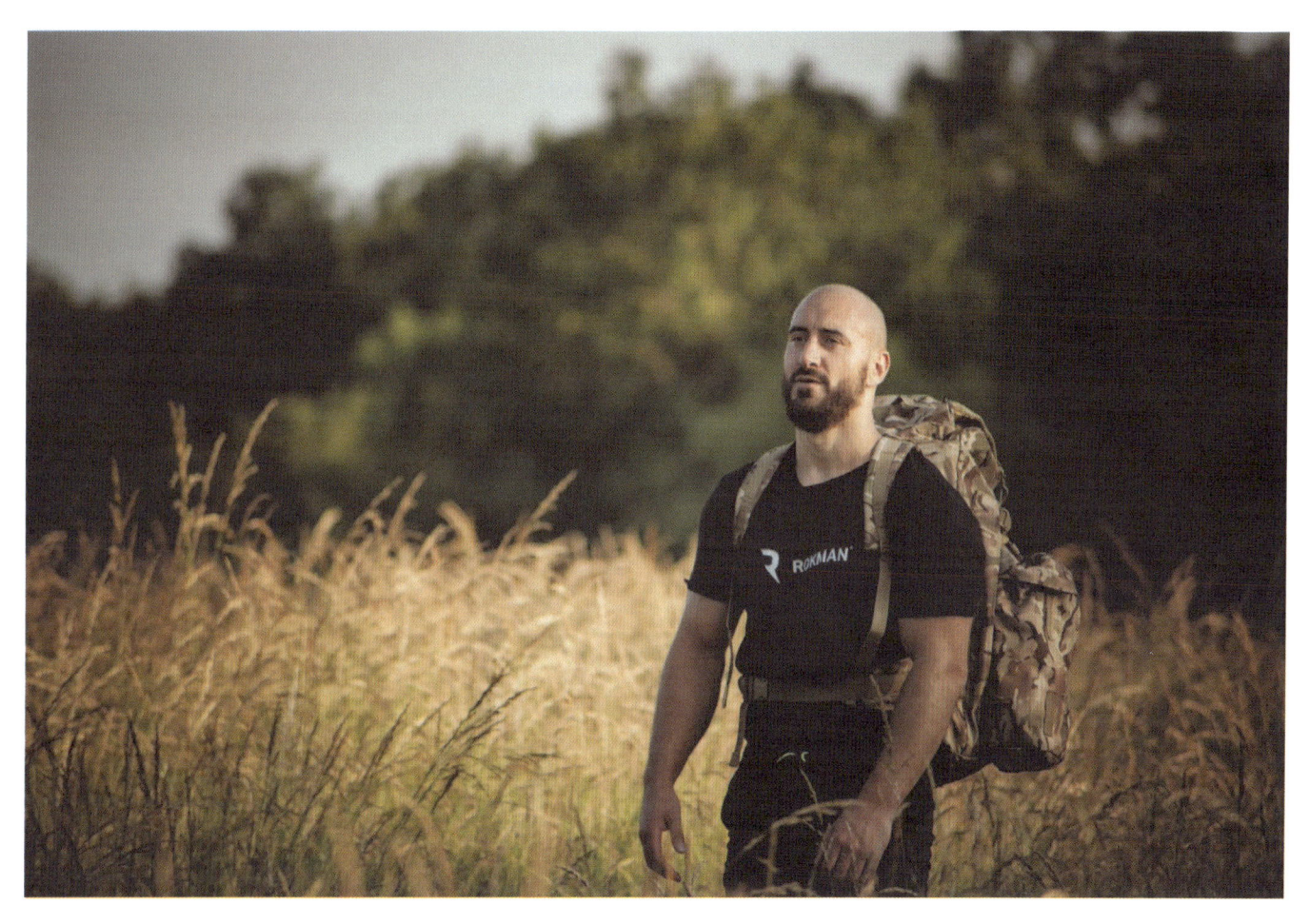

Max Glover is a fitness enthusiast who now enjoys writing about his extreme challenges. The former Royal Marine has led a varied and unique life previously working as a maritime security operative and close protection officer and is now a proud ambassador of the mental resilience and running brand Rokman.

With stories to tell and training programmes to write - Max has pushed himself to the limits through a variety of disciplines - running, bodybuilding and calisthenics. Most recently raising thousands of pounds for charity by towing an 18-tonne truck for 2 miles (Furthest known distance), carrying a piano up a mountain, carrying 100kg for 100km (furthest known distance) and towing a 1.7 tonne car for 26.2 miles (smashing the world record at the time).

Max spends his down time relaxing with his family and cats and is most happy these days rucking with a heavy Bergen (military rucksack) enjoying the great outdoors... and is looking forward to sharing his next adventure with you!

More books from Max Glover:

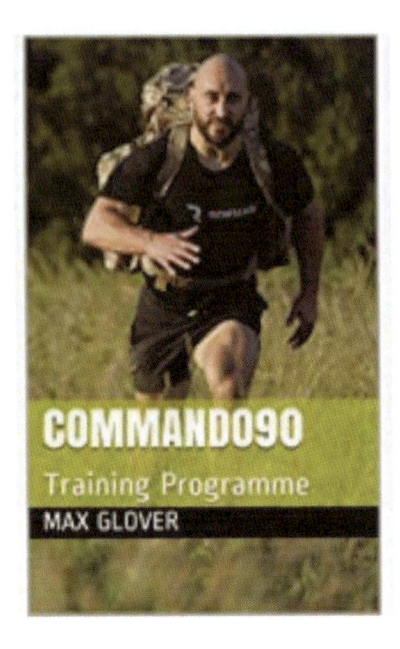

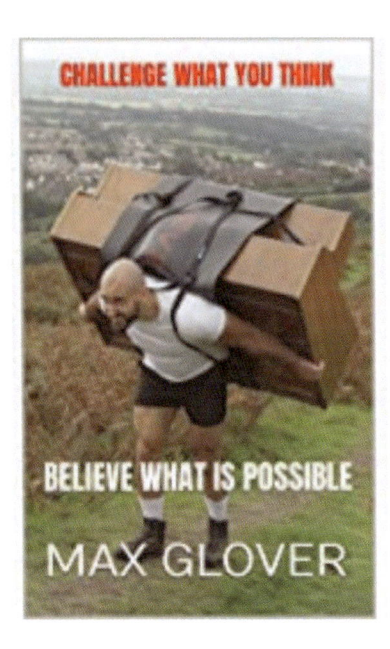

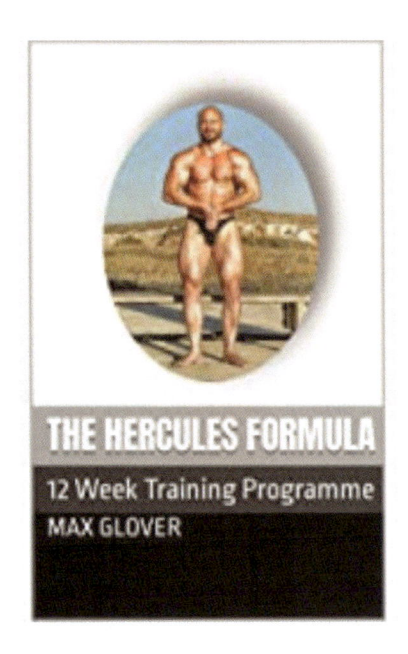

Commando90 – a 90 day no BS guide to obtain a Commando level of fitness. This is raw and basic, suitable for those who just want to follow a guide without any unnecessary distractions. Intense circuit training sessions for different abilities. Can be completed with bodyweight only and no fancy gym equipment.

Challenge What You Think, Believe What is Possible – Max Glover lets you into his mind while he completes unique challenges, such as carrying a piano up a mountain, towing a car for a marathon and much more. He explains how he trained for each challenge and also valuable lessons and insights from his time in the Royal Marines.

The Hercules Formula – This is a 12 week bodybuilding programme with the sole purpose of getting bigger and stronger using weights.

Image credits: Rokman www.rokman.co.uk @teamrokman
www.maxglover.com
Instagram: @muscle.world.fitness

If you have bought the book, please feel free to leave me some feedback and let me know how you got on!

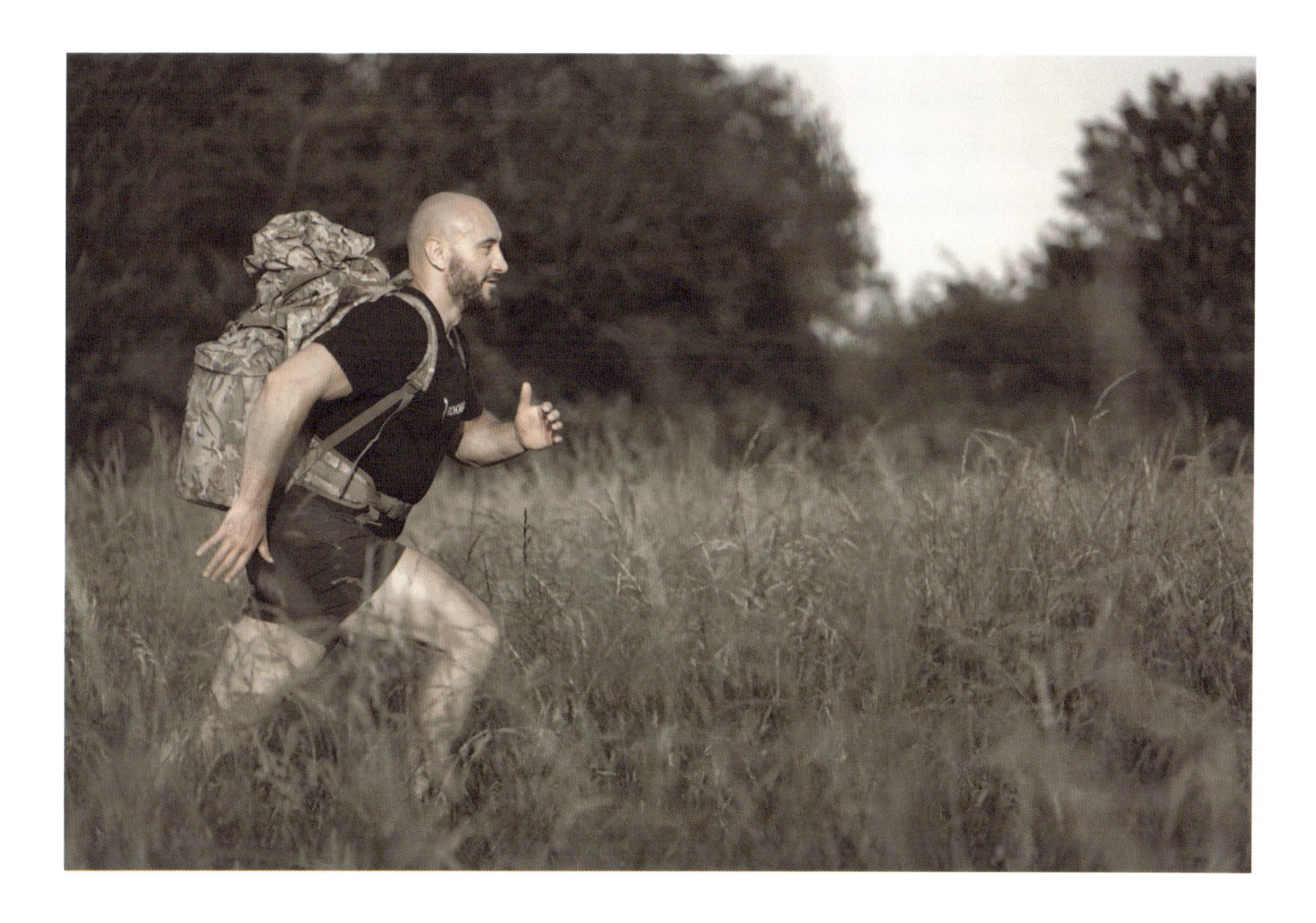

COMMANDO

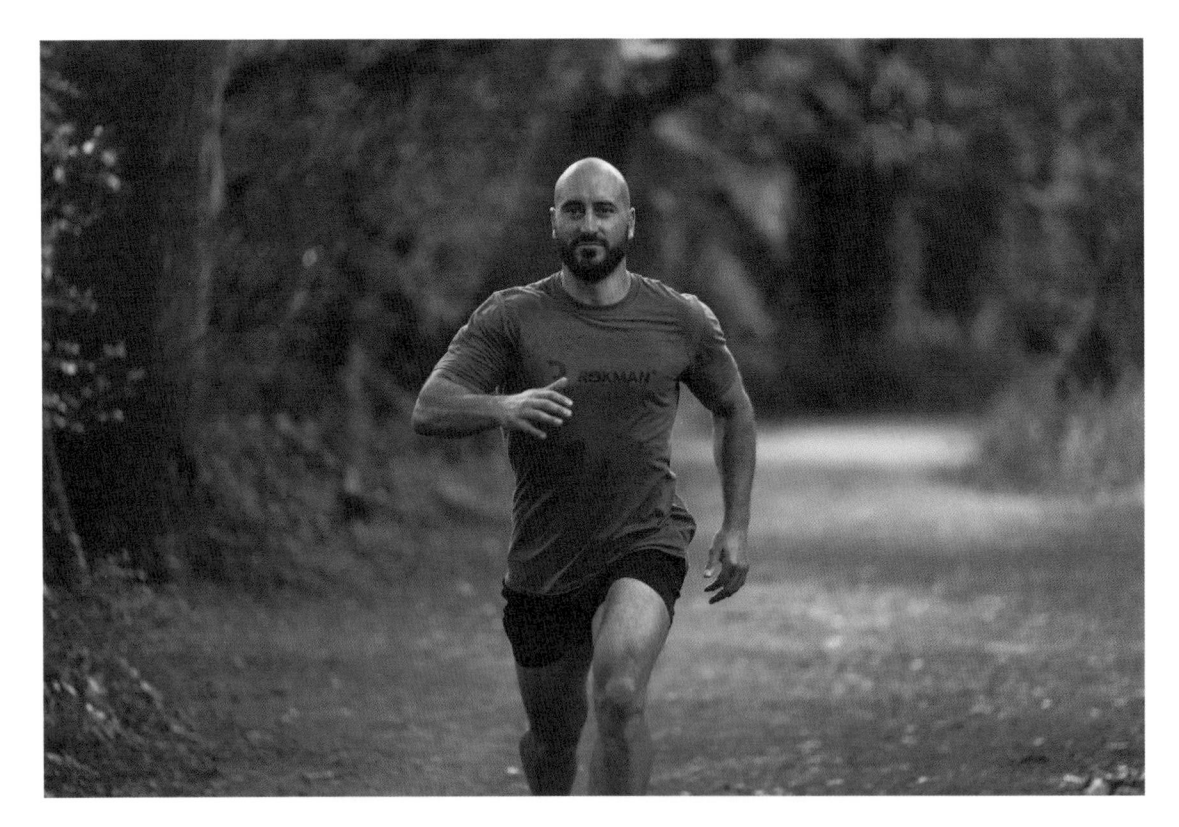

RUNNER

Max Glover

Printed in Great Britain
by Amazon